CURRENT TOPICS IN ANESTHESIOLOGY

Edited by **Riza Hakan Erbay**

Current Topics in Anesthesiology
http://dx.doi.org/10.5772/63140
Edited by Riza Hakan Erbay

Contributors

Zeki Tuncel Tekgül, Burcu Özalp Horsanalı, Mustafa Ozan Horsanali, Jesse Musokota Mumba, Freddy Kasandji Kabambi, Christian Tshebeletso Ngaka, Ayse Belin Ozer, Sibel Ozcan, Takashi Kawano, Fabricio Locatelli, İsmail Demirel, Esef Bolat, Aysun Yıldız Altun, Yusuke Asakura, Maho Kinoshita, Yusuke Kasuya, Makoto Ozaki, Yuta Matsunaga, Masahiko Tsuchiya

Published by InTech

Janeza Trdine 9, 51000 Rijeka, Croatia

Publishing Process Manager Iva Simcic

Technical Editor SPi Global

Cover InTech Design team

First published February, 2017

Printed in Croatia

Additional hard copies can be obtained from orders@intechopen.com

Current Topics in Anesthesiology, Edited by Riza Hakan Erbay

p. cm.

Print ISBN 978-953-51-2917-2

Online ISBN 978-953-51-2918-9

For EU product safety concerns:
IN TECH d.o.o., Prolaz Marije Krucifikse Kozulić 3, 51000 Rijeka, Croatia,
info@intechopen.com or visit our website at intechopen.com.

Meet the editor

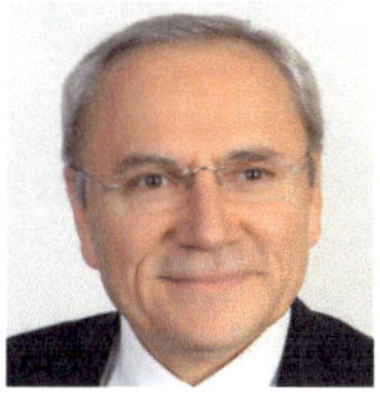

Prof. Dr. Riza Hakan Erbay became an anesthesiologist at the Pamukkale University in 1996. He obtained his titles of assistant professor in 1997, associate professor in 2005, and professor in 2011. He has mainly worked in the field of orthopedic anesthesia, regional anesthesia, and intensive care medicine. He worked as an education coordinator in the Faculty of Medicine during 2007–2009. He served as the vice president of Surgical Sciences Department of Faculty of Medicine during 2009–2012. He obtained the title of intensivist in 2013. He worked as a head of the Anesthesiology Clinic in Izmir Tepecik Training and Research Hospital during 2013–2014. He is currently the chairman of Department of Anesthesiology and Reanimation at the Faculty of Medicine of the Pamukkale University.

Contents

Preface

Anesthesiology is a science that has progressively evolved due to viable technological improvements and thriving accumulation of knowledge within the very extensive and explorable nature of itself. Consequently, the enhanced knowledge and technological availability have played major parts in terms of upgrading and changing the clinical applications. The more effective and reliable drugs are introduced in the practice of anesthesiology day by day; also, the use of ultrasonography is rapidly advancing toward the routine. On the other hand, although the healthcare policies of the nations have some restriction on healthcare resources, the concepts of efficient resource utilization and healthcare quality standards also provide some improvements in the practice. This book provides contemporary knowledge about local anesthetics and their pharmacology and toxic effects of anesthetic drugs in children. Also, this book includes some new technological developments in the use of ultrasonography in regional anesthesia as well as some contemporary topics in anesthesiology. I am grateful to the authors for their contributions to this book, and I wish it will be helpful to the readers.

Prof. Dr. Riza Hakan Erbay
Chairman of Department of Anesthesiology and Reanimation
Faculty of Medicine, Pamukkale University
Denizli, Turkey

Section 1

Local Anesthetics

Chapter 1

Pharmacology of Local Anaesthetics and Commonly Used Recipes in Clinical Practice

Jesse Musokota Mumba,
Freddy Kasandji Kabambi and
Christian Tshebeletso Ngaka

Additional information is available at the end of the chapter

http://dx.doi.org/10.5772/67048

Abstract

Local anaesthetics are commonly used drugs in clinical anaesthesia. The knowledge of their pharmacology is paramount for safe and optimal use of this group of drugs. This chapter consists of two sections. The first section will address the chemical and physical properties, pharmacokinetics and pharmacodynamics of the local anaesthetics. In the second section, examples of the commonly used doses and additives used for various peripheral and regional anaesthetics will be discussed. We will also address the treatment of toxicity as a result of inadvertent intravascular injection of the local anaesthetics.

Keywords: local anaesthetics, lidocaine, bupivacaine, ropivacaine, cocaine

Summary points

1. Local anaesthetics block the transmission of pain from the nerve endings into the central nervous system. Chemically, they are classified as esters and amides depending on the intermediate chain between the lipophilic aromatic ring and the hydrophilic amine group.
2. The primary mode of action is blockade of the fast voltage-gated sodium channels. To achieve this effect, the unionised fraction of the drug crosses the lipid bilayer of the axoplasm and blocks the channel intracellularly.
3. The duration and density of the block depend on both the volume and concentration of the agent used.

4. Factors that influence the efficacy of local anaesthetics are the pH, pKa, lipid solubility, protein binding and the length of the intermediate chain. Efficacy can be augmented by use of adjuncts such as adrenaline, opioids, alpha 2-adrenergic agonists (clonidine) and alkalinisation.
5. Toxicity is related to the site of injection, the vascularity of the site and the injected dose. The use of vasoconstrictors may reduce toxicity due to reduction in systemic absorption.
6. From the local anaesthetics in clinical use, racemic bupivacaine has the highest affinity for the sodium channels and is the most difficult to manage in the event of systemic toxicity.

1. The neuron and pharmacology of local anaesthetics

1.1. Introduction

Local anaesthetics are drugs that block conduction of electrical impulses in excitable tissues. These tissues include the nerve cells and myocytes (both cardiac and skeletal muscles). Analgesia and anaesthesia occur as a result of the blockage of electrical impulses. Other local anaesthetics like lidocaine also possess Class I antiarrhythmic properties. Before a detailed venture into the physical-chemical properties and mechanism of action of this class of drugs, a brief overview of the nerve anatomy is discussed. This will aid in the overall understanding of how these agents work and how their efficacy and safety can be improved by the use of appropriate doses and adjuncts.

1.2. Nerve anatomy

Neurons are the primary cells in the nervous system. The nervous system is made up of the central and peripheral nervous system. It can also be looked at in terms of parasympathetic and sympathetic nervous system. A group of neurons bundled together make up *peripheral nerves*. The basic structure of a neuron is illustrated in **Figure 1**.

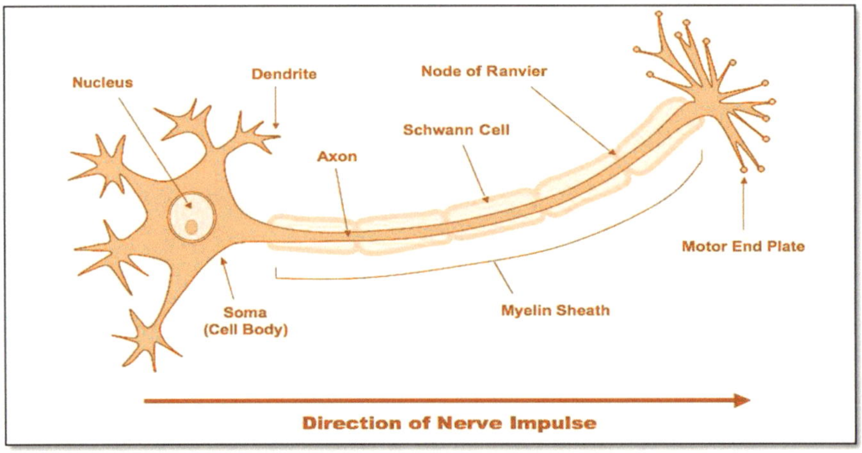

Figure 1. Structure of a neuron. Source: http://www.vce.bioninja.com.au/aos-2-detecting-and-respond/coordination--regulation/nervous-system.html. Used with permission 05/11/2016.

Peripheral nerves contain both afferent and efferent fibres, which are bundled into one or more fascicles as illustrated in **Figure 2**. Individual nerve fibres within the fascicle are surrounded by a layer of loose connective tissue called the endoneurium. The endoneurium houses the glial cells, fibroblasts and blood vessel capillaries, all of which are integral to the function of the nerve fibre. The fascicle is in turn surrounded by a dense layer of collagenous connective tissue called the perineurium. A cylindrical sheath called the epineurium forms the outermost layer of a peripheral nerve. The main function of these layers is to protect the nerve fibres and also act as barriers to agents acting on the nerves including local anaesthetics.

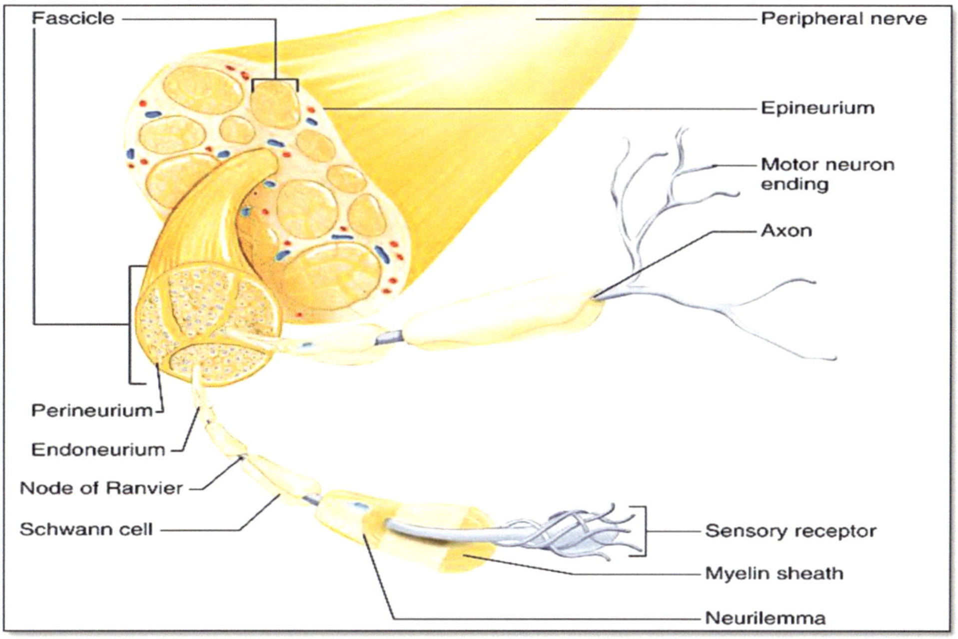

Figure 2. Peripheral nerve. Source: https://www.studyblue.com/#flashcard/review/8819508.

1.3. Electrophysiology of nerve conduction

The resting membrane potential of a nerve cell is in the range of −60 to −70 mV. At rest, neurons are more permeable to potassium ions due to the presence of potassium leak channels. This explains why the resting neuronal membrane potential is closer to the equilibrium potential of potassium of −80 mV. The ionic disequilibria acts as the energy needed for propagation of action potentials on the cell surface [1]. The intracellular milieu of the nerve cell is negatively charged relative to the extracellular. Upon excitation of the nerve fibres, the electrical impulse propagates along the axon as a result of changes occurring in the adjacent membrane alternating from negative to positive values of about +50 mV due to rapid influx of sodium ions. At an electrical potential of +50 mV, there is rapid efflux of potassium ions in an attempt to maintain electrical neutrality of the cell. To restore the resting membrane potential, the sodium/potassium ATPase pumps sodium extracellularly, while the opposite happens to the potassium ions. The conduction of impulses along nerve fibres occurs as small brief, localised spikes of depolarisation on the surface of the cell membrane. Impulses travel in one direction as the axonal membrane that has just undergone depolarisation remains in the refractory state until the resting potential is restored by the Sodium/Potassium ATPass pumps on [2]. **Figure 3** illustrates the sequence of events occurring during the propagation of the action potential.

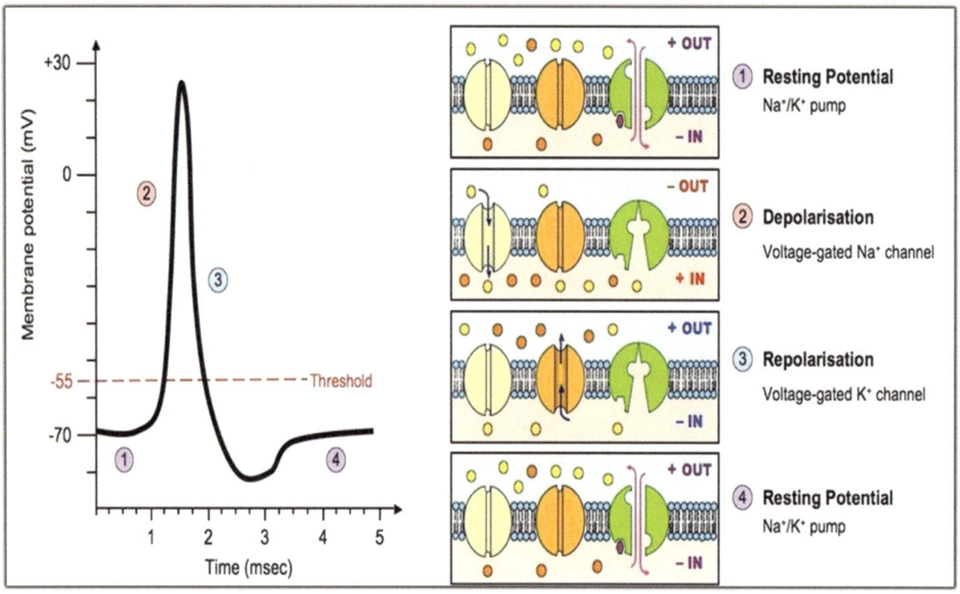

Figure 3. Sequence of events occurring during the propagation of the action potential. Source: http://www.vce.bioninja.com.au/aos-2-detecting-and-respond/coordination--regulation/nervous-system.html. Used with permission 05/11/2016.

1.4. Pharmacology of local anaesthetics

1.4.1. Structure-activity relationship of local anaesthetics

Local anaesthetics consist of a hydrophilic amine and a lipophilic aromatic ring connected by an intermediate chain. The structural bond in the intermediate chain determines whether the local anaesthetic will be classified as an ester or an amide. Furthermore, the bond in the intermediate chain determines the pathway of metabolism of the compound. Ester local anaesthetics are metabolised by plasma pseudocholinesterases, whereas the amides are metabolised in the liver by the cytochrome family of enzymes.

Figure 4 illustrates the structure of an ester and amide local anaesthetic showing clearly the bonds in the intermediate chains.

http://dx.doi.org/10.5772/67048

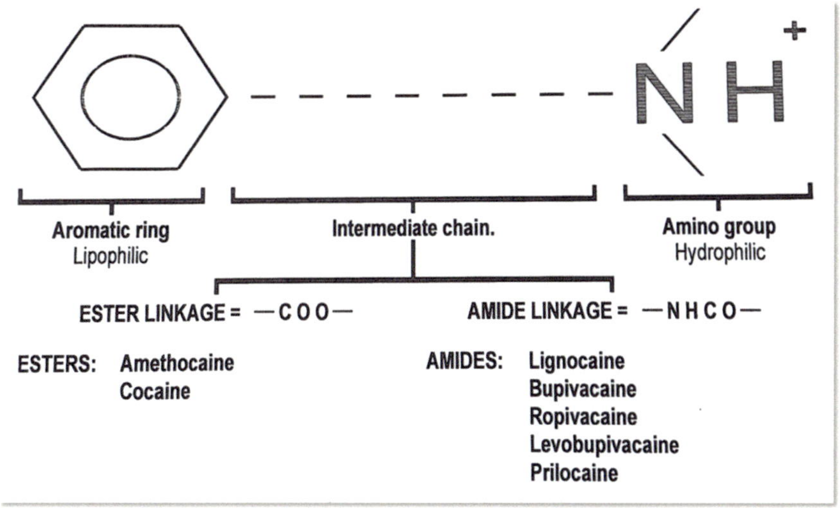

Figure 4. The structure of an ester and amide local anaesthetic showing clearly the bonds in the intermediate chains. Source: Student's Manual, Department of Anaesthesia and Perioperative Medicine. University of Cape Town, South Africa. Used with permission, 16/11/2016.

1.4.2. Mechanism of action of local anaesthetics

Local anaesthetic blocks the transmission of nerve impulses by reversibly blocking the fast voltage-gated sodium channels, thereby inducing analgesia and anaesthesia. Physicochemically, local anaesthetics are weak bases that are formulated in an acidic milieu, hence containing a larger proportion of the drug in the ionised state. However, it is the unionised fraction that is able to cross the lipid bilayer neuronal membrane and block the voltage-gated sodium channels from the inside of the axoplasm. This blockade renders the sodium channel inactive, and hence, no further conduction of impulses occurs. Diagramatically this is well demonstrated by **Figure 5**.

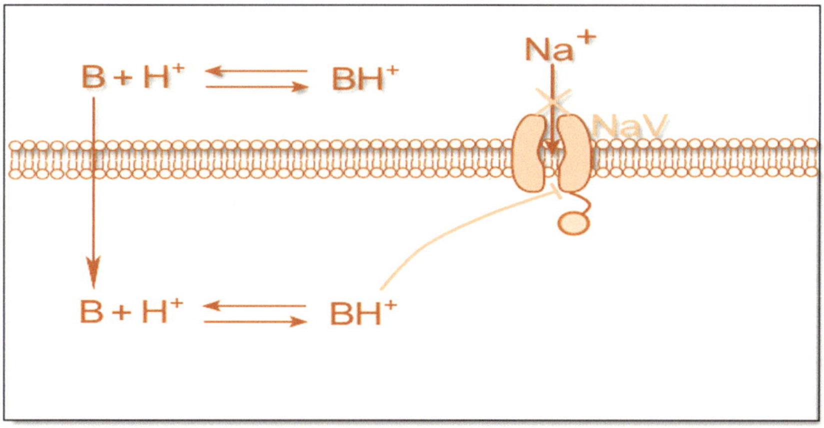

Figure 5. Mechanism of action of local anaesthetics. Source: http://www.esciencecentral.org/ebooks/minimally-invasive/anesthesia-cosmetic-procedures.php. Used with permission 05/11/2016.

1.4.3. Determinants of physiological activities of local anaesthetics

The activity of local anaesthetics is influenced by a number of factors. These include the pH of the surrounding tissue, the lipid solubility of the local anaesthetic, pKa, the bond in the intermediate chain and its length and the protein binding of the particular local anaesthetic in question. Details of how each of these factors influence the activity of local anaesthetics is discussed below:

1. pKa: The pKa is the pH at which the number of ionised and unionised fractions of the drug is in equilibrium. *The lower the pKa, the* more the unionised fraction is present for any given pH and hence *the faster the onset of action.*

2. pH: *The lower the pH, that is, acidic milieu, the less the potency because in* acidic conditions the ionised fraction predominates, there is less of the unionised fraction, and there is less of the local anaesthetic available to cross the lipid bilayer and block the voltage-gated sodium channels. This explains why local anaesthetic does not have much efficacy in reducing pain in infected tissues like abscesses in which the pH of such tissues is much lower than the physiological pH of 7.4.

3. Lipid solubility: The more lipid soluble the local anaesthetic is, the higher the potency, the faster the onset of action and the longer the duration of action. This is because there are more drug molecules able to cross the lipid bilayer of the neuronal membrane and create a 'depot' of the drug from within the axoplasm.

4. Intermediate chain: The longer the intermediate chain, the more potent the local anaesthetic. Bupivacaine has a longer intermediate chain compared to lidocaine. Bupivacaine is three to four times more potent than lidocaine.

5. Protein binding: Local anaesthetics with higher degrees of protein binding have longer duration of action.

Depending on the type of nerves and their fibres, the sequence of blockade of the nerve fibres is illustrated in **Table 1**.

Fibre type	Myelin	Diameter (μm)	Function	Conduction velocity	Onset of block
A-α	Yes	12–20	Somatic motor and proprioception	Fast	Slow
A-β	Yes	5–12	Light touch and pressure	↓	↓
A-γ	Yes	3–6	Muscle spindle (stretch)		
A-δ	Yes	1–4	Firm touch, pain (fast-localising) and temperature		
B	Yes	1–3	Preganglionic autonomic		
C	No	0.3–1.3	Pain (nonlocalising ache), temperature, touch, postganglionic autonomic	Slow	Fast

Table 1. Classification of nerve fibres and sequence of blockade.

http://dx.doi.org/10.5772/67048

1.5. Specific local anaesthetics

As discussed above, local anaesthetics are classified as ester and amides. Amethocaine also known as tetracaine and cocaine is the ester of clinical importance.

Cocaine was first introduced into clinical practice in 1884. It was first used in ophthalmic surgery and later in dental surgery. Currently, it is mainly used topically in ear, nose and throat (ENT) surgeries at a concentration of 4–10%. The onset of action is fast and lasts 20–30 min. Due to its ability to sensitise adrenergic receptors, it is relatively contraindicated in patients known with hypertension and ischaemic heart diseases. Concurrent use of adrenaline is contraindicated because cocaine is a potent vasoconstrictor.

Amethocaine (tetracaine) is another ester used widely in clinical practice. It was introduced in 1930 for ophthalmics/ophthalmology and as a cream for use to locally anaesthetise venepuncture sites, especially in the paediatric population. The onset of action is relatively fast with a long duration of action. A maximum dose of 1 mg/kg is recommended. It is the least metabolised of ester local anaesthetics and hence possesses a higher risk of toxicity. Other ester local anaesthetics in use include benzocaine, prilocaine and 2-chloroprocaine.

Some of the amide local anaesthetics exhibit isomerism. Previously, sold drugs were racemic mixtures containing both the levo and dextro enantiomers. The levorotatory enantiomers of local anaesthetics are typically less neural and cardiotoxic than dextrorotatory enantiomers. For this reason, most clinicians had a preference/opted for pure enantiomers. With the introduction of better monitoring and ultrasound-guided blocks, the racemic mixtures are making their way back into clinical practice as they tend to have a longer duration of action [3].

Lidocaine was the first amid local anaesthetics to be introduced in 1948. It remains one of the most widely used anaesthetics as it can be used intravenously, intrathecally and as a local infiltration. It is also a Class 1b antiarrhythmic drug. It has a fast onset of action due to its pKa of 7.8, which is closer to the physiological pH of 7.4, and is moderately water and lipid soluble. It has a moderate duration of action and is the least toxic of all amides probably due to its relatively low protein-binding capacity of 64%. The addition of adrenaline, a vasoconstrictor, reduces its toxicity allowing for higher doses to be used for local tissue infiltrations. The recommended doses are 3 mg/kg without adrenaline and 7 mg/kg with adrenaline, respectively. Concerns have been raised over neurotoxicity with lidocaine making it much less popular in recent years for intrathecal usage. For localised procedures such as hand surgeries, 0.5% lidocaine intravenously post-exsanguination of the limb is still a widely used technique introduced by August Biers in 1908.

Mepivacaine is an intermediate duration of action compared to lidocaine and bupivacaine. It was introduced in 1957. It has a pK_a of 7.6. It has similar pharmacokinetic and dynamic properties with lidocaine except for some concerns of it being neurotoxic in the neonate. However, its properties of low rates of systemic toxicity, rapid onset and dense motor block make mepivacaine attractive for procedures such as shoulder surgery.

Ropivacaine was introduced in 1976. It has a pK_a of 8.2. Its chemical structure is similar to both mepivacaine and bupivacaine. Ropivacaine is available as a pure levorotatory stereoisomer only. It is a pure enantiomer and less cardiotoxic compared with racemic mixtures of other local anaesthetics. With respect to its better safety profile, ropivacaine has become a preferred long-acting local anaesthetic for peripheral nerve block anaesthesia for many providers. The motor block sparing properties associated with ropivacaine spinal and epidural analgesia may provide an advantage over bupivacaine. Despite its safety profile, all standard precautions pertaining to use of local anaesthetics are encouraged as they have been incidences of cardiovascular collapse reported with its use [4].

Bupivacaine exists as levo and dextro enantiomer. Its racemic form was introduced in 1963, while levobupivacaine was introduced in 1995. It has a pK_a of 8.1 and a protein binding of 96%. The higher degree of protein binding makes bupivacaine the longest acting and most cardiotoxic local anaesthetic if inadvertently administered intravenously. It has been used successfully over the years since its introduction and has become the yardstick for all other long-acting local anaesthetics. Interestingly, at low concentration, bupivacaine has the propensity for sensory blocks while mildly sparing the motor blocks (differential sensitivity). This property allows for 'walking epidural' in labour analgesia. The maximum recommended dose is 2 mg/kg with or without adrenaline as there is only a modest increase in the duration of action when combined with a vasoconstrictor. It is three to four times more potent than lidocaine, but the onset of action is much slower.

2. Local anaesthetic toxicity: what factors affect the presentation of toxicity and management of toxicity

Local anaesthetic toxicity can be observed at local tissue level and systemically. The systemic toxicity of local anaesthetic depends on plasma concentration which in itself is closely related to the dose and the site of injection. We, the authors, will first discuss local tissue toxicity and thereafter expand on the clinical manifestation of the systemic toxicity.

2.1. Local tissue toxicity

2.1.1. Local anaesthetic-induced neurotoxicity

Local anaesthetics exert a direct time and dose-dependant toxicity on neurons and myocytes. The mere injection of local anaesthetics perineurally or intrathecally is a risk factor for perioperative nerve injury. Local anaesthetic-induced nerve injury may occur at clinical concentration levels when accidentally injected intrafascicularly. In an experimental model, axonal degeneration has been noticed in such instances [5].

Some local anaesthetics are packaged in concentration much higher than used in clinical practice. Care should be taken to prepare a safe dilution to reduce the risk of nerve toxicity. The outer layer of connective tissue surrounding the nerve fibre, the perineurium, forms the 'blood-nerve barrier' and protects the nerve from chemical injury. The correct dilution of local anaesthetics will ensure that the concentration in the perineural and intraneural milieu is within the therapeutic range, thereby avoiding neural damage. The use of adjuncts to increase the viscosity of the solution also has been associated with increased incidence of nerve injury.

The use of hyperbaric solution in continuous spinal anaesthesia cases leads to the pooling of the solution in the caudal dural sac and prolongs the toxic effect on the nerve fibres (i.e. cauda equina syndrome) [6]. Transient neurologic syndrome after a single bolus of lignocaine for spinal anaesthesia has been reported as well, though with a good outcome in the short term [7]. Lignocaine seems more prone to cause local anaesthetic neurotoxicity than bupivacaine with risk of 6.5 as high as bupivacaine probably due to the former's lower pKa, and hence, more unionised drug crosses into the axoplasm [8].

2.1.2. Incidence and risk factors

The true incidence of local anaesthetic-induced neurotoxicity is difficult to account for as there are many confounding risk factors in the perioperative period that can lead to nerve injury. Large prospective studies have shown that the overall incidence of neurologic complication with peripheral nerve block technique is <3%. Most of these complications are transient sensory deficits [9, 10]. The risk factors pertaining to neurotoxicity will further be grouped as anaesthetic factors, surgical factors and patient factors.

1. **Anaesthetic factors**

(a) Peripheral nerve blocking is an independent risk factor for local anaesthetic neurotoxicity [11].

(b) The site of injection of local anaesthetics. More claims of neurotoxicity have been tabled after brachial plexus block than other blocks, after intrafascicular than extrafascicular injection as the earlier directly exposes the nerve fibre to high concentration of local anaesthetics [12, 13].

2. **Surgical risk factors**

The use of tourniquet to reduce blood loss and provide favourable operative field causes compression of nerve fibre and tissue ischaemia which has synergetic effect as far as local anaesthetic neurotoxicity is concerned. Furthermore, the vasa nervorum is compressed by tourniquet use, and the washout of local anaesthetic is reduced, thereby prolonging the exposure of nerve fibre to local anaesthesia.

3. **Patient risk factors**

(a) Pre-existing neuropathies: diabetic peripheral neuropathy, Guillain-Barre syndrome and multiple sclerosis all put the nerve fibre at increased risk of local anaesthetic-induced neurotoxicity.

(b) Peripheral vascular diseases: vasculitis, smoking and hypertension affect the microvasculature and therefore may make nerves more vulnerable to ischaemia and increased risk of neurotoxicity of local anaesthetics during the perioperative period.

2.1.3. Pathophysiology

The mechanism of this neurotoxicity at a cellular level is not well elucidated. The postulated mechanisms involve the intrinsic caspase pathway, the phosphoinositide 3-kinase (PI3K) pathway and the mitogen-activated protein kinase (MAPK) pathway, but there is no consensus on what the predominant pathway may be [14, 15]. The interaction of the local anaesthetic and the voltage-gated sodium channel (VGSC) and G-coupled protein receptors is unlikely to be the pathophysiological pathway through which local anaesthetics exert their neurotoxicity. A study using tetrodotoxin, another sodium channel blocker, does not support that hypothesis [16].

2.1.4. Local anaesthetic-induced muscle toxicity

Local anaesthetics cause muscle damage after intramuscular injection. The effect is more pronounced with potent and long-acting local anaesthetic like bupivacaine. These effects on skeletal muscle are transient and with full recovery within 2 weeks.

The tissue toxicity may also be the result of preservative used to maintain stability of drug molecules in solution. Sodium bisulphite and ethylene glycol tetra acetic acid are thought to be the culprits for the neurotoxicity of chloroprocaine.

2.2. Systemic toxicity

Systemic toxicity from local anaesthetics is closely related to the systemic concentration achieved either through excessive dose or inadvertent intravascular injection of local anaesthetics. The cardiovascular system and central nervous system are the most affected systems, the latter being more sensitive than the former. This entails that the local anaesthetic blood concentration required to produce the toxic sign and symptoms is lower for the CNS than for the cardiovascular system (CVS). This translates in clinical practice as the appearance of signs and symptoms of CNS toxicity first, followed by those of the CVS. However, caution needs to be exercised here as when a patient is having a conscious sedation or a full general anaesthetic, the CNS toxicity may be masked and the cardiotoxicity in the form of cardiovascular collapse may be the only manifestation of the local anaesthetic toxicity. The main risk factors for developing systemic toxicity are:

- extremes of age (younger than 4 months or older than 79 years)
- pre-existing heart conduction abnormality
- ischaemic heart disease
- renal dysfunction
- hepatic dysfunction
- pregnant women
- injection at a highly vascular site (e.g. intercostal block).

2.2.1. Central nervous system toxicity

The signs and symptoms of central nervous system toxicity are generally classified into two distinct phases, the excitatory phase and the depression phase, respectively.

2.2.1.1. *The excitatory phase*

The earliest symptom is usually the metallic taste, followed by circumoral numbness, light-headedness, dizziness, visual disturbances, disorientation, tinnitus and agitation. During this period, signs of toxicity include shivering, muscular twitching, tremor and generalised tonic-clonic convulsion. The generally accepted explanation for this sequence of events is that the inhibitory neurons are the first to be blocked by local anaesthetics leaving the activity of the excitatory neurons unopposed [17].

2.2.1.2. *The depression phase*

The muscle twitches and convulsion subsides, followed by respiratory depression and respiratory arrest. The respiratory depression will lead to hypoventilation and raised plasma pCO_2 and a state of respiratory acidosis which will potentiate the CNS toxicity of local anaesthetics [18]. The explanation for this increased CNS toxicity relies on the fact that raised plasma CO_2 level increases its diffusion into the cell, therefore decreasing the intracellular pH. The acidic intracellular environment will favour the conversion of the unionised local anaesthetics to the ionised form, which will be unable to diffuse out of the cell leading to a phenomenon known as ion trapping. Decreased plasma binding of local anaesthetics [19] and increased cerebral blood flow contribute to the increased delivery of local anaesthetics to the brain, and this too increases the likelihood of CNS toxicity.

The clinician needs to be aware of these facts as they will influence the approach to management of the CNS toxicity of local anaesthetics.

2.2.2. *Cardiovascular system toxicity*

The effect of local anaesthetics on the cardiovascular system is direct and indirect. They affect the heart directly through the decrease in the rate of depolarisation of conducting cell and cardiomyocytes secondary to the block of voltage-gated sodium channel. There is a decrease in the duration of action potential and refractory period [20, 21]. Various local anaesthetics have a different degree of disruption of the conduction of action potential through the heart. Bupivacaine depresses the conduction to a greater degree than lignocaine. It produces cardiovascular toxicity at a lower concentration than that of lignocaine and has a worse outcome after cardiac resuscitation. However, ropivacaine and levobupivacaine, a pure S-enantiomer of bupivacaine, do not share this tendency for greater cardiac toxicity [22].

A raised plasma level of local anaesthetics first prolongs the duration of conduction in the atrium and ventricle noticed on an electrocardiogram as PR interval prolongation and QRS complex widening. The spontaneous pacemaker activity is depressed at a higher plasma level resulting in bradycardia and sinus arrest successively. Ventricular arrhythmia occurs more often with bupivacaine than lignocaine, with an increased risk in pregnant patients. Apart from conduction disturbance, local anaesthetics also have a negative inotropic activity [23] on the heart through interference with sarcolemmal sodium and calcium channel activities [24].

Low concentration of local anaesthetics causes vasoconstriction, and higher concentration causes vasodilation with the exception of cocaine, which consistently produces vasoconstriction regardless of the concentration [21].

2.2.3. *Management of local anaesthetic toxicity*

The management of cardiovascular toxicity is based on sound understanding and implementation of the basic principle of cardiopulmonary resuscitation [25]. The steps for effective management of CNS toxicity of local anaesthetics include:

- Stop injection or infusion of the agent.
- Call for help and start basic life support.
- Airway management: administer 100% O_2 to prevent hypoxaemia, ventilate the patient to prevent hypercarbia, and acidosis which potentiate the CNS toxicity of local anaesthetics [20]. Ensure the patency of airway: if the patency of the airway is compromised or patient is unable to maintain the airway, securing the airway endotracheal tube and subsequent ventilation is recommended.
- Suppress seizures with the use of benzodiazepines or induction of a full general anaesthesia.
- In case of a cardiovascular collapse, effective chest compression as per the advanced cardiac life support (ACLS) guideline should commence. Clinicians need to be aware that CPR in a setting of local anaesthetics cardiac toxicity will require prolonged effort and dosage adjustment (limit epinephrine bolus doses to <1 mcg/kg which is far less than in a classic CPR protocol).
- Avoid vasopressin, calcium channel blockers, beta blockers or local anaesthetic in the management of cardiac arrhythmia.
- Twenty per cent of intralipid should be used without delay along with the initial resuscitative measures as per the practice guidelines of the American Society of Regional Anaesthesia (ASRA) [25].
- A bolus of 1.5 mL/kg IV for 1 min followed by an infusion of 0.25 mL/kg/min.
- Repeat bolus once or twice for persistent cardiovascular collapse.
- Double the infusion rate to 0.5 mL/kg/min if blood pressure remains low.
- Continue infusion for at least 10 min after attaining circulatory stability.
- Recommended upper limit: approximately 10 mL/kg lipid emulsion over the first 30 min.

2.3. Methaemoglobinemia

This is a complication associated with a specific local anaesthetic, namely prilocaine. Prilocaine is metabolised in the liver, and o-toluidine is produced as a by-product of this metabolism.

O-toluidine is a strong oxidant that oxidises haemoglobin to methaemoglobin. Severe methaemoglobinemia can be treated effectively with an infusion of methylene blue [21].

3. Commonly used Adjuvants to local anaesthetics in clinical practice

Local anaesthetics added to the number of anaesthetic techniques to accommodate various patient groups depending on the type of surgery and patient's functional status. Amide local anaesthetics (LA) are the most widely used in modern clinical anaesthetic practice. However, Anaesthesiologists still awaits development of an ideal LA with longer duration of action, better nerve fibre selectivity, a lesser degree of motor blockade and lower incidences of systemic toxicity. In this quest, multiple adjuvants have been used in clinical practice with varying results. This section aims to discuss the adjuvants to LA for nerve blocks, spinal anaesthesia, caudals and epidural anaesthesia. The actual techniques and complications are beyond the scope of this chapter.

3.1. Adjuvants to local anaesthetics (LA)

1. Opioids

The use of neuraxial opioids in human subjects dates back to 1979 [26, 27]. Since then, they have been proven to provide effective and prolonged analgesia [28]. In addition, this synergy allows for decreased LA doses with the hope to reduce the incidence of hypotension for similar pain relief. Combining LA with intrathecal morphine has been shown to prolong analgesic effect after lower limb arthroplasty and spinal anaesthesia [29–31]. Epidural opioids also provide similar analgesic benefit although only limited to 6 h following joint arthroplasty [32]. These benefits have to be balanced against a high incidence of side effects including respiratory depression (which may be delayed up to several hours post-administration), nausea, vomiting and urinary retention [33]. The evidence for analgesic benefit of using opioids in brachial plexus blocks over systemic administration is scanty [34].

Fentanyl has a more rapid onset and shorter duration of action in comparison with more hydrophilic opioids such as morphine when administered neuraxially. The recommended intrathecal dose is 10–25 μg, and the epidural loading dose is 50–100 μg. It does not prolong motor block thus allowing for early ambulation. The duration of action is 2–4 h, and the risk of respiratory depression is very low and of short duration.

Morphine: a hydrophilic drug less readily absorbed in the spinal cord resulting in slower onset but prolonged duration of analgesia, and as it moves cephalad via CSF, the analgesia spreads over more dermatomes. However, this late cephalad spread increases the potential for brainstem binding and delayed respiratory depression although very rare in clinical practice. The recommended dose is 50–300 μg intrathecal and 2–5 mg epidural loading dose. The risk of side effects increases exponentially with the increase in the dose.

Diamorphine: a diacetylated analogue of morphine with a potency of approximately 1.5–2 times that of morphine resulting in a faster onset and slightly shorter duration of action. The intrathecal dose is 300–400 μg, and epidural loading dose is 2–3 mg.

Sufentanil: an intrathecal dose is 2.5–10 μg, and epidural loading dose is 10–50 μg. It is an extremely potent opioid with a faster onset of action. Its use in clinical practice is limited by its short duration of action and high side effect profile.

2. Alpha-2 adrenoceptor agonists

Clonidine: intrathecal use of clonidine as an adjunct to local anaesthetics prolongs the duration of sensory blockade by approximately 1 h [35]. However, the duration of motor blockade is increased, and the incidence of hypotension is also high. The recommended dose for intrathecal use is in the range of 15–150 μg with the incidence of adverse effects (bradycardia, sedation, hypotension) increasing with doses above 150 μg. In paediatric anaesthesia, the use of clonidine (1 mg/kg) for caudal blocks doubles the duration of analgesia when compared to LA alone, but causes sedation. Further research is needed to examine the benefits of using clonidine for peripheral nerve and plexus blocks [36].

Dexmedetomidine is a highly selective alpha-2 adrenoceptor agonist. There is some evidence to suggest a clinical benefit to use of dexmedetomidine with LA for intravenous regional anaesthesia [37].

Adrenaline has direct and indirect actions as an adjuvant. It acts directly on α-2 adrenoceptors in the substantia gelatinosa of the dorsal horn of the spinal cord resulting in presynaptic inhibition of transmitter release from C and Aδ fibres. Indirectly, it causes local vasculature constriction thus prolonging the duration of action of the LA. Adrenaline used as an adjunct to thoracic epidural infusions improves the quality of analgesia [38, 39]. There are conflicting reports regarding the use of adrenaline in lumbar epidurals.

3. *N*-methyl-d-aspartate receptor antagonists

Ketamine: preservative-free ketamine injected into the caudal epidural space for children at a dose of 0.5 mg/kg has been shown to extend analgesia time by several hours. The opponents of ketamine cite increased the risk of psychotomimetic side effects, but the use of benzodiazepine premedication prior to block reduces the risk of these side effects.

Magnesium: intrathecal or epidural magnesium has been used with variable results. It may prolong LA/opioid block in women in labour at a dose of 50 mg, but a very high dose of magnesium has been reported to produce transient neurological toxicity.

4. Other adjuvants

Other adjuvants like midazolam and neostigmine have been suggested to improve the quality of analgesia. However, the high incidence of significant side effects far outweighs the small improvement in analgesia.

4. Commonly used recipes in clinical practice

1. Spinal anaesthesia (SA) for caesarean delivery

The ideal subarachnoid dose of local anaesthesia for caesarean delivery has been debated for a long time. Most anaesthetists employ hyperbaric 0.5% bupivacaine in a dose of 7.5–15.0 mg. A meta-analysis suggests any reduction in the bupivacaine dose during single-shot SA to less than 8 mg with opioid or 10 mg alone, resulting in a significantly increased requirement for analgesic

http://dx.doi.org/10.5772/67048

supplementation and possibly conversion to general anaesthesia [40]. The practice at our institution is to use 10 mg of hyperbaric bupivacaine plus 10 μg fentanyl with satisfactory results.

2. Labour epidural analgesia

The current policy at our institution is to draw up a mixture of 5 mL of 0.5% bupivacaine, 4 mL saline and 50 μg fentanyl, that is, a total of 10 mL of 0.25% bupivacaine with 5 μg/mL fentanyl, and to administer two 4 mL boluses of this mixture 3 min apart, with the patient in the left lateral position for the first bolus and the right lateral for the second. In early labour, an initial bolus of 8 mL of 0.125% bupivacaine may be given, followed by a repeat dose of a similar volume. The aim is to obtain levels of T8–T10 bilaterally, and this can take up to 20 min. Analgesia is maintained with an infusion of 0.125% bupivacaine plus 2 μg/mL fentanyl at the rate of 8–14 mL/h.

Top-up of labour epidural for caesarean delivery step-by-step

- Draw up 17 mL 2% lignocaine, plus 50 μg fentanyl, 1 mL 8.4% sodium bicarbonate and 1 mL 1/10,000 adrenaline (i.e. 1 mL of an ampoule which has been diluted 10 times). This makes a total of 20 mL, with approximately 1/200,000 adrenaline.
- Administer 5 mL boluses after a test dose.
- Unless the initial dose of epidural bupivacaine has been administered within the previous hour, treat as though the patient has no block at all. Most patients will require between 16 and 22 mL for an effective block to T4.
- Conversion to spinal anaesthesia may result in a high block if there has been an unsuccessful attempt at a top-up with a large volume of local anaesthetic.
- A poorly functioning epidural catheter is best re-sited, or spinal anaesthesia may be performed using a reduced dose (unpredictable), or general anaesthesia may be preferred.

3. Local anaesthetics for regional intravenous anaesthesia

Regional intravenous anaesthesia is indicated for short operative procedures for extremities and sometimes for pain therapy (e.g. treatment of complex regional pain syndromes). This is a very basic technique, and it requires 12–15 mL of 2% lidocaine or 30–40 mL of 0.5% lidocaine for upper extremity regional anaesthesia. Other local anaesthetics such as bupivacaine are contraindicated for IV injection for reasons discussed in the toxicity section. Some evidence exits supporting a better quality of the block by use if additives such as ketamine and alpha-2 agonists are added to local anaesthetics for peripheral nerve blocks [41, 42].

Equipment required includes:

- Lidocaine
- IV cannulae
- Double pneumatic tourniquet
- Esmarch bandage
- Syringes

Technique:

- An IV cannula is inserted in the extremity opposite the block side.
- A double pneumatic tourniquet is placed with proximal cuff high on the upper arm.
- A peripheral IV cannula is placed on the limbs on which surgery is to be done as distal as feasible
- The block arm is elevated for 1–2 min to allow passive exsanguination, and then, Esmarch bandage is wrapped around the arm to exsanguinate the extremity completely.
- The distal cuff is inflated to 50–100 mmHg above systolic BP after which the proximal cuff is inflated followed by deflation the distal cuff.
- Inject preservative-free local anaesthetic (recommended maximum dose is 3 mg/kg).
- After injection IV cannula is removed from anaesthetised hand and pressure is quickly applied to puncture site.
- Anaesthesia onset is almost immediate.
- When the patient reports tourniquet pain inflate the distal cuff and deflate the proximal cuff.

4. Local anaesthetics for peripheral nerve blocks

There are a wide variety of local anaesthetic agents available for peripheral nerve blocks. Important points to consider when making the choice are onset and duration of action, duration of the surgical procedure and anticipated degree of pain. Caution is to be used if one decided to use additives to local anaesthetics for peripheral nerve blocks to prolong their effect as none of the additives discussed in this chapter have got the Food and Drug Administration (FDA) approval for this purpose [43].

5. Topical anaesthetics

Topical anaesthetics are used for procedures such as vein cannulation, laceration repair to avoid infiltrative local anaesthesia injections and associated pain. They are widely used in the paediatric population. There are many dosage forms in clinical use, for example, gels, sprays, creams, ointments, patches. Skin absorption is variable and accounts for the systemic toxicity. This complication is rare provided the skin is intact with the exception of 5% EMLA cream, a eutectic mixture of 2.5% lidocaine and 2.5% prilocaine. Commonly available forms are Ametop (4% tetracaine) and EMLA, and more recently, a 4% lidocaine topical cream has been introduced. It is better tolerated on the skin while having flexible application times. Onset of action for Ametop is between 30 and 40 min and has a duration of action of about 4–5 h. EMLA on the other hand has a slower onset of about 60 min with a short duration of action of about 2 h. Toxicity is largely related to the age of the patients and possible damage in the skin. It is recommended that in those below 3 months, duration of application should not be more than 1 h, while for age group between 3 and 12 months maximum duration of application does not exceed 4 h [44].

6. Neuraxial techniques in paediatrics

Caudal anaesthesia is a popular technique to provide analgesia in paediatric patients. The single-shot technique is often adequate for most urological, lower extremity and lower abdominal procedures. An indwelling catheter can extend its use to upper abdomen and thoracic procedures and offers the added benefit of continuous post-operative analgesia. The LA dose depends on the operative site that ranges from 0.5 to 2 mL/kg of 0.25% bupivacaine, that is, the level of the block is proportional to the dose.

Spinal and epidural anaesthesia are safe and effective ways to provide anaesthesia for infants [45]. For spinal anaesthesia, bupivacaine 0.5% at a dose 0.5–1 mg/kg is commonly used with the dose decreasing with increasing age.

Local anaesthetics add to the armament that is at the disposal of anaesthetists. Understanding of their pharmacology increases the safety with which these drugs can be used. Early recognition of toxicity is core to avoiding central nervous system and cardiorespiratory collapse.

Author details

Jesse Musokota Mumba[1*], Freddy Kasandji Kabambi[2] and Christian Tshebeletso Ngaka[2]

*Address all correspondence to: jesse@jesmuira.com

1 Head of Anaesthesia and Critical Care, Ondangwa Private Hospital, Namibia

2 Department of Anaesthesia and Perioperative Medicine, University of Cape Town, South Africa

References

[1] Hodgkin, A. L., & Katz, B. (1949). The effect of sodium ions on the electrical activity of the giant axon of the squid. The Journal of Physiology, 108(1), 37–77.

[2] Hodgkin, A. L., & Huxley, A. F. (1952). A quantitative description of membrane current and its application to conduction and excitation in nerve. The Journal of Physiology, 117(4), 500–544.

[3] Paul Barash, Bruce F. Cullen, Robert K. Stoelting, Michael Cahalan, Christine M. Stock, Rafael Ortega. (2013). Clinical anesthesia, 7th ed. Lippincott Williams & Wilkins. pp. 561–579. Ch 21. ISBN 978-1-4511-4419-2

[4] Litz, R. J., Popp, M., Stehr, S. N., & Koch, T. (2006). Successful resuscitation of a patient with ropivacaine-induced asystole after axillary plexus block using lipid infusion*. Anaesthesia, 61, 800–801. doi:10.1111/j.1365-2044.2006.04740

[5] Selander, D., Brattsand, R., Lundborg, G., Nordborg, C., Olsson, Y. (1979). Local anesthetics: importance of mode of application, concentration and adrenaline for the appearance of nerve lesions. An experimental study of axonal degeneration and barrier damage after intrafascicular injection or topical application of bupivacaine (Marcain). Acta Anaesthesiologica Scandinavica, 23(2), 127–136.

[6] Rigler, M. L., Drasner, K., Krejcie, T. C., Yelich, S. J., Scholnick, F. T., DeFontes, J., et al. (1991). Cauda equina syndrome after continuous spinal anesthesia. Anesthesia & Analgesia, 72(3), 275–281.

[7] Pollock, J. E. (2003). Neurotoxicity of intrathecal local anaesthetics and transient neurological symptoms. Best Practice & Research Clinical Anaesthesiology, 17(3), 471–484.

[8] Eberhart, L. H., Morin, A. M., Kranke, P., Geldner, G., Wulf, H. (2002) Transient neurologic symptoms after spinal anesthesia. A quantitative systematic overview (meta-analysis) of randomized controlled studies. Anaesthesist. 51(7), 539–546.

[9] Auroy, Y., Narchi, P., Messiah, A., Litt, L., Rouvier, B., Samii, K. (1997). Serious complications related to regional anesthesia: results of a prospective survey in France. Anesthesiology, 87(3), 479–486.

[10] Nouette-Gaulain, K., Capdevila, X., Rossignol, R. (2012). Local anesthetic 'in-situ' toxicity during peripheral nerve blocks: update on mechanisms and prevention. Current Opinion in Anesthesiology, 25(5), 589–595.

[11] Welch, M. B., Brummett, C. M., Welch, T. D., Tremper, K. K., Shanks, A. M., Guglani P., et al. (2009). Perioperative peripheral nerve injuries: a retrospective study of 380,680 cases during a 10-year period at a single institution. Anesthesiology, 111(3), 490–497.

[12] Brull, R., McCartney, C. J., Chan, V. W., El-Beheiry, H. (2007). Neurological complications after regional anesthesia: contemporary estimates of risk. Anesthesia & Analgesia, 104(4), 965–974.

[13] Brull, R., Hadzic, A., Reina, M. A., Barrington, M. J. (2015). Pathophysiology and etiology of nerve injury following peripheral nerve blockade. Regional Anesthesia and Pain Medicine, 40(5), 479–490.

[14] Lirk, P., Haller, I., Myers, R. R., Klimaschewski, L., Kau, Y. C., Hung, Y. C., et al. (2006). Mitigation of direct neurotoxic effects of lidocaine and amitriptyline by inhibition of p38 mitogen-activated protein kinase in vitro and in vivo. Anesthesiology, 104(6), 1266–1273.

[15] Hogan, Q. H. (2008). Pathophysiology of peripheral nerve injury during regional anesthesia. Regional Anesthesia and Pain Medicine, 33(5), 435–441.

[16] Sakura, S., Bollen, A. W., Ciriales, R., Drasner, K. (1995). Local anesthetic neurotoxicity does not result from blockade of voltage-gated sodium channels. Anesthesia & Analgesia, 81(2), 338–346.

[17] Wagman, I. H., De Jong, R. H., Prince, D. A. (1967). Effects of lidocaine on the central nervous system. Anesthesiology, 28(1), 155–172.

[18] Englesson, S., Grevsten, S. (1974). The influence of acid-base changes on central nervous system toxicity of local anaesthetic agents. II. Acta Anaesthesiologica Scandinavica, 18(2):88–103.

[19] Burney, R. G., DiFazio, C. A., Foster, J. A. (1978). Effects of pH on protein binding of lidocaine. Anesthesia & Analgesia, 57(4), 478–480.

[20] Englesson, S. (1974). The influence of acid-base changes on central nervous system toxicity of local anaesthetic agents. I. An experimental study in cats. Acta Anaesthesiologica Scandinavica, 18(2), 79–87.

[21] Miller, Ronald D. Miller's Anesthesia. 7th ed. Philadelphia, PA: Churchill Livingstone/ Elsevier, 2010. Vol. 1. pp 913-940. Ch. 30. ISBN: 978-0-4430-6959-8

[22] Feldman, H. S., Arthur, G. R., Pitkanen, M., Hurley, R., Doucette, A. M., Covino, B. G. (1991). Treatment of acute systemic toxicity after the rapid intravenous injection of ropivacaine and bupivacaine in the conscious dog. Anesthesia & Analgesia, 73(4), 373–384.

[23] Block, A., Covino, B. G. (1981). Effect of local anesthetic agents on cardiac conduction and contractility. Regional Anesthesia and Pain Medicine, 6(2), 55–61.

[24] Chamberlain, B. K., Volpe, P., Fleischer, S. (1984). Inhibition of calcium-induced calcium release from purified cardiac sarcoplasmic reticulum vesicles. Journal of Biological Chemistry, 259(12), 7547–7553.

[25] Neal, J. M., Mulroy, M. F., Weinberg, G. L., American Society of Regional A, Pain, M. (2012). American Society of Regional Anesthesia and Pain Medicine checklist for managing local anesthetic systemic toxicity: 2012 version. Regional Anesthesia and Pain Medicine, 37(1), 16–18.

[26] Behar, M., Magora, F., Olshwang, D., Davidson, J. T. (1979). Epidural morphine in treatment of pain. Lancet. 1979, 1(8115), 527–529.

[27] Wang JK, Nauss LA, Thomas JE. Pain relief by intrathecally applied morphine in man. Anesthesiology. 1979 Feb;50(2):149–51

[28] Morgan, M. The rational use of intrathecal and extradural opioids. British Journal of Anaesthesia, 63(2), 165–188.

[29] Fischer, H. B. J., Simanski, C. J. P., Kehlet, H., et al. (2005). A procedure-specific systematic review and consensus recommendations for analgesia after total hip replacement. Anaesthesia, 60(12),1189–1202.

[30] Fischer, H. B. J., Simanski, C. J. P., Sharp, C., et al. (2008). A procedure-specific systematic review and consensus recommendations for postoperative analgesia following total knee arthroplasty. Anaesthesia, 63(10), 1105–1123.

[31] Dahl, J. B., Jeppesen, I. S., Jørgensen, H., Wetterslev, J., Møiniche, S. (1999). Intraoperative and postoperative analgesic efficacy and adverse effects of intrathecal opioids in patients undergoing cesarean section with spinal anesthesia. Anesthesiology, 91(6), 1919.

[32] Choi, P. T., Bhandari, M., Scott, J., Douketis, J. (2003). Epidural analgesia for pain relief following hip or knee replacement. Cochrane Database of Systematic Reviews. 3:CD003071.

[33] Chaney, M.A. (1995). Side effects of intrathecal and epidural opioids. Canadian Journal of Anesthesia, 42(10), 891–903.

[34] Murphy, D. B., McCartney, C. J., Chan, V. W. (2000). Novel analgesic adjuncts for brachial plexus block: a systematic review. Anesthesia & Analgesia, 90(5), 1122–1128.

[35] Elia, N., Culebras, X., Mazza, C., Schiffer, E., Tramèr, M. R. (2008). Clonidine as an adjuvant to intrathecal local anesthetics for surgery: systematic review of randomized trials. Regional Anesthesia and Pain Medicine, 33(2), 159–167.

[36] Pöpping, D. M., Elia, N., Marret, E., Wenk, M., Tramèr, M. R. (2009). Clonidine as an adjuvant to local anesthetics for peripheral nerve and plexus blocks: a meta-analysis of randomized trials. Anesthesiology, 111, 406–415.

[37] Esmaoglu, A., Mizrak, A., Akin, A., Turk, Y., Boyaci, A. (2005). Addition of dexmedetomidine to lidocaine for intravenous regional anaesthesia. European Journal of Anaesthesiology, 22(6), 447–451.

[38] Sakaguchi, Y., Sakura, S., Shinzawa, M., Saito, Y. (2000). Does adrenaline improve epidural bupivacaine and fentanyl analgesia after abdominal surgery? Anaesth Intensive Care, 28(5), 522–526.

[39] Niemi, G., Breivik, H. (1998). Adrenaline markedly improves thoracic epidural analgesia produced by a low-dose infusion of bupivacaine, fentanyl and adrenaline after major surgery. A randomised, double-blind, cross-over study with and without adrenaline. Acta Anaesthesiologica Scandinavica, 42(8), 897–909.

[40] Arzola, C., Wieczorek, P. M. (2011). Efficacy of low-dose bupivacaine in spinal anaesthesia for Caesarean delivery: systematic review and meta-analysis. British Journal of Anaesthesia, 107(3), 308–318.

[41] Brown, E. M., McGriff, J. T., Malinowski, R. W. (1989). Intravenous regional anaesthesia (Bier block): review of 20 years' experience. Canadian Journal of Anesthesia, 36, 307–310.

[42] Kumar, A., Sharma, D., Datta, B. (2012). Addition of ketamine or dexmedetomidine to lignocaine in intravenous regional anesthesia: a randomized controlled study. Journal of Anaesthesiology, Clinical Pharmacology, 28(4), 501–504. doi:10.4103/0970-9185.101941

[43] Kirksey, M. A., Haskins, S. C., Cheng, J., Liu, S. S. (2015). Local anesthetic peripheral nerve block adjuvants for prolongation of analgesia: a systematic qualitative review (Schwentner C, ed). PLoS One, 10(9), e0137312. doi:10.1371/journal.pone.0137312

[44] Fraczek, M., Demidas, A. (2012). Acta Assessment of the efficacy of topical anesthetics using the tactile spatial resolution method. Acta Dermatovenerologica Croatica, 20, 7–13.

[45] Williams, R. K., Adams, D. C., Aladjem, E. V., et al. (2006). The safety and efficacy of spinal anesthesia for surgery in infants: the vermont infant spinal registry. Anesthesia & Analgesia, 102(1), 67–71.

Section 2

A Novel Monitoring in Ultrasonography

Chapter 2

Regional Anesthesia: Advantages of Combined Use with General Anesthesia and Useful Tips for Improving Nerve Block Technique with Ultrasound Technology

Masahiko Tsuchiya

Additional information is available at the end of the chapter

http://dx.doi.org/10.5772/66573

Abstract

Regional anesthesia is not always performed independently, but rather is frequently employed as part of a general anesthesia technique. Thus, its procedures and usefulness should be considered in settings where general anesthesia is used. In this chapter, new perspectives regarding the interaction of regional and general anesthesia are presented, as well as novel tips for improving nerve block techniques during the course of general anesthesia, Regional anesthetics inhibit superoxide generation of neutrophils by inhibition of protein kinase C activity and also have potent antioxidant activities, while inhalation general anesthetics have contrasting effects. Therefore, it is considered that regional anesthetics are able to compensate for shortcomings of inhalation general anesthetics by reducing surgical oxidative stress. In clinical settings, combined use of regional with general anesthesia provides better intraoperative hemodynamics than general anesthesia alone, particularly in high-risk patients affected by severe cardiovascular disease. To further improve the analgesic potency and duration of regional anesthesia, especially in cases in which a peripheral nerve block is performed, addition of low molecular weight dextran as an adjuvant to the local anesthetic solution is quite effective. Furthermore, recent advancements in ultrasound technology have made previously difficult regional anesthesia techniques easier and safer to achieve. A typical example is use of a caudal block in adults, which is quite difficult with a conventional method. Expanding its indication to adults is beneficial, especially for high-risk patients undergoing surgery in the lower abdomen. Furthermore, proper in-line positioning of ultrasound images is key for successful and easy completion of ultrasound-guided procedures, such as needle insertion to the target. We have been able to establish such a positioning method by use of an iPad and the VT-100 image transfer system (Scalar Co., Tokyo, Japan). Following consideration of the present findings and related experience, it is evident that performance of regional anesthesia under general anesthesia provides great advantages, including better and safe anesthesia management.

Keywords: regional anesthesia, antioxidant activity, neutrophils, AAPH, Phycoerythrin, protein kinase C, ultrasound-guided nerve block, transversus abdominis plane block, intraoperative hemodynamics, caudal block, adjuvant, low molecular weight dextran, iPad, wireless image transmission, image position, radial artery catheterization

1. Introduction

With recent advancements in ultrasound technology, nerve block procedures have become easier and their accuracy improved [1, 2]. As a result, many regional anesthetic methods and techniques previously overlooked have been reevaluated, which has led to recent increased interest among anesthesiologists, with large numbers of papers and textbooks concerning regional anesthesia published during the past 10 years. However, the interrelationship between regional and general anesthesia has not been well-elucidated. Regional anesthesia is not always performed as an independent procedure in daily practice; rather it is frequently included as part of a general anesthesia technique, thus a full understanding of its effects is important to evaluate usefulness in settings where general anesthesia is employed. In the present chapter, new perspectives regarding the interaction of regional anesthesia with general anesthesia as well as the use of ultrasound technology are discussed based on findings obtained by our research team. Discussions regarding the antioxidant activities of local anesthetics and their effects for stabilizing the hemodynamics of patients under general anesthesia, the best adjuvants for local anesthetics used for regional nerve block, a simple but important tip for improving the accuracy and easiness of ultrasound-guided procedures, and other related topics are included.

2. Oxidative stress associated with surgery and inhalation anesthetics

Although the possibility that surgery increases oxidative stress has been suggested for several years [3, 4], how it develops remains unclear, especially during surgery. Analysis of intraoperative changes in the ferric-reducing ability of plasma may lead to a breakthrough for elucidation of surgical oxidative stress, as the reduction of ferric irons to ferrous irons in plasma is a simple but sensitive indicator of the antioxidant potential of blood in clinical settings [5]. These changes can be measured by use of a biological antioxidant power (BAP) test with an FRAS 4 analyzer (Wismerll Co. Ltd. Tokyo, Japan), which is based on color changes of a solution containing a source of ferric ions adequately bound to a special chromogenic substrate at 505 nm when the ferric ions are reduced to ferrous ions according to antioxidant activity induced by addition of plasma.

Using this unique method, adult patients with ASA I-II who underwent an open colectomy with sevoflurane anesthesia along with fentanyl and vecuronium were investigated. During surgery, the ferric reducing ability was significantly lowered, indicating that the colectomy procedure increased oxidative stress resulting in a reduction in the antioxidant ability of blood (**Figure 1**). To the best of our knowledge, these are the first reported findings to clearly demonstrate that surgery increases oxidative stress.

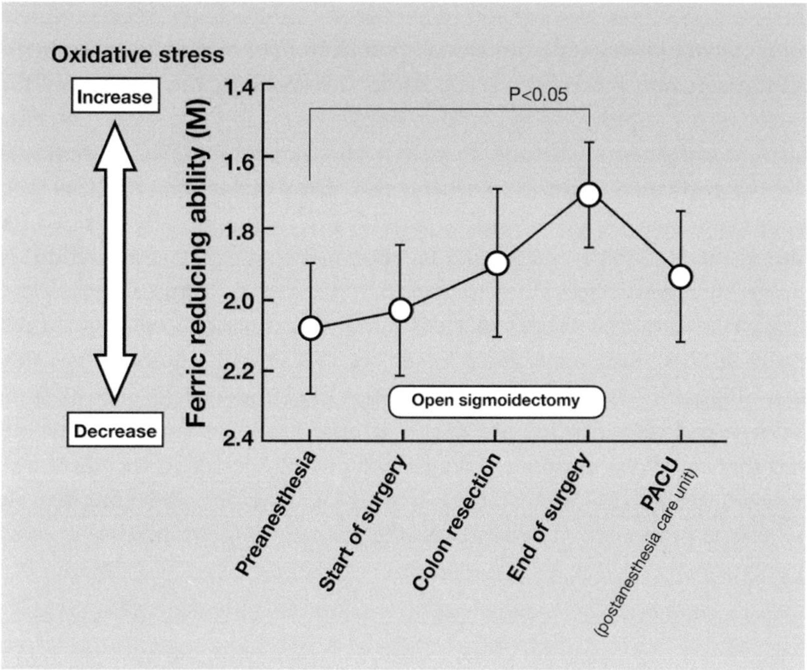

Figure 1. Plasma ferric-reducing ability in 18 patients who underwent an open sigmoidectomy with sevoflurane anesthesia. Lower values indicate increased oxidative stress; thus, our findings demonstrated that surgery increases oxidative stress.

Oxidative stress may also be a key factor to determine patient surgical stress [5], and we investigated this issue in cases of cardiac surgery [6]. Preoperative oxidative stress was determined by measuring plasma hydroperoxide values using a d-Rom test with an FRAS 4 analyzer, while the occurrence of major organ morbidity and mortality (MOMM) was also assessed. MOMM included death, deep sternal infection, reoperation, stroke, renal failure requiring hemodialysis, and prolonged ventilation (>48 h). Our results showed that an elevated preoperative hydroperoxide level in cardiac surgery patients is an independent risk factor for severe postoperative complications, and its reliability to predict postoperative complications appeared to be better as compared to preoperative BNP values and the European system for cardiac operative risk evaluation (EuroSCORE). The optimal threshold value of hydroperoxide concentration to differentiate between patients with and without MOMM was found to be 450 UCarr (sensitivity, 87.0%; specificity, 81.9%). These findings indicated that preoperative oxidative stress is an important risk factor for postoperative complications. In addition, they suggested the therapeutic potential of antioxidant therapy in surgical patients, as antioxidant control may reduce surgical stress, thereby improving postoperative recovery.

On the other hand, the drug used for inhalation anesthesia also has an oxidant effect. We studied the effects of inhalation anesthetics on protein kinase C (PKC) activity, which has been implicated in regulation of cell secretion, modulation of membrane conductance, release of neurotransmitters, regulation of cytoplasmic Ca^{2+}, functional modification of receptors, and other components of the signal transduction machinery [7–9]. As for neutrophils, the ability of PKC activators such as TPA to trigger superoxide generation suggests a role for protein phosphorylation in the mechanism of transmembrane signaling. In addition, purified PKC stimulates superoxide generation by the particulate fraction of neutrophils. Thus, activation of PKC is involved in the process of superoxide generation of neutrophils [10, 11]. Using partially purified PKC from rat brains, we found that halothane, a typical inhalation anesthetic [12], activated this enzyme and increased superoxide generation from neutrophils (**Figure 2**). Furthermore, other inhalation anesthetics have been reported to activate PKC in a similar manner according to their anesthetic potency (**Figure 3**) [7–9]. H-7, a specific inhibitor of PKC, totally inhibited halothane-induced PKC activation (**Figure 4**) and superoxide generation of neutrophils (**Figure 2**), confirming that the reaction developed via activation of PKC [9]. In addition to the findings in blood cells, it has been reported that sevoflurane, another typical inhalation anesthetic, increases the generation of reactive oxygen species (ROS) in isolated hearts [13]. Together, these findings strongly suggest negative effects of inhalation general anesthetics including an increase in oxidative stress in surgical patients.

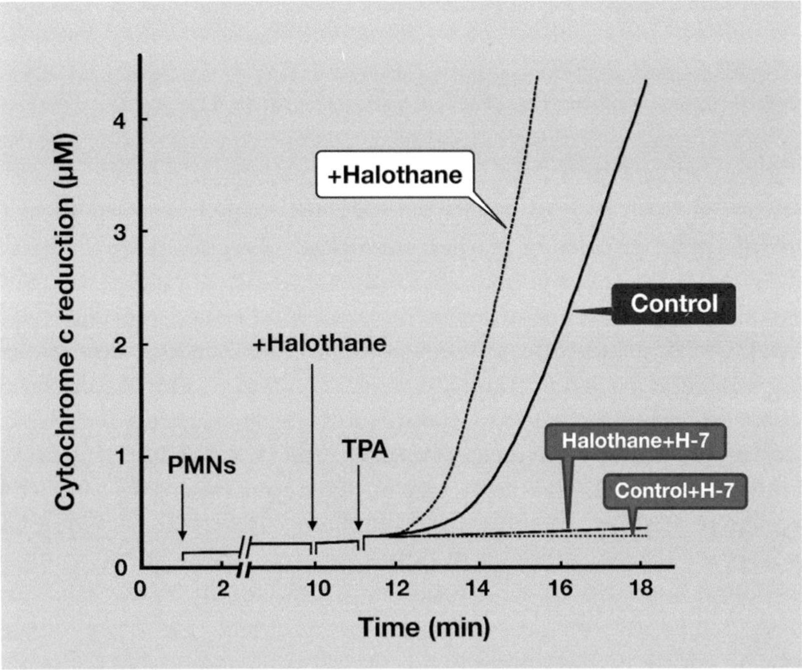

Figure 2. Effects of halothane and H-7 (l-(5-isoquinolinesulfonyl) methylpiperazine dihydrochloride) on superoxide generation by neutrophils. Superoxide generation was spectrophotometrically analyzed by measuring the reduction of cytochrome c at 550 nm with a reference wavelength of 540 nm. Neutrophils were obtained from a guinea pig using a method previously described [10], then 2×10^6 cells·ml^{-1} were incubated in KRP (Krebs-Ringer phosphate solution) medium containing 1 mM Ca^{2+}, 10 mM glucose, 25 μM cytochrome c, and 0.1 mM NaN_3 at 37°C. The concentrations of halothane, TPA (12-O-tetradecanoylphorbol-13-acetate), and H-7 were 0.59 mM, 0.4 nM, and 100 μM, respectively. Halothane activated superoxide generation by neutrophils, whereas H-7, a specific inhibitor of protein kinase c, inhibited that activation.

http://dx.doi.org/10.5772/66573

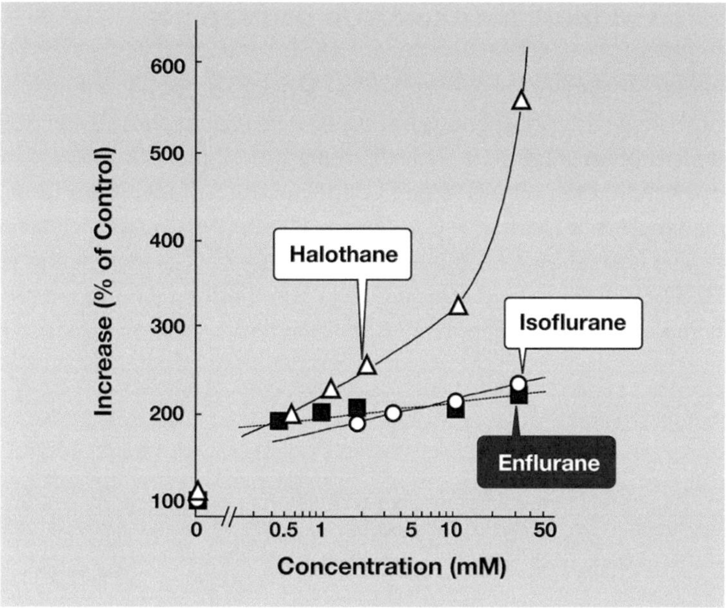

Figure 3. Effects of inhalation anesthetics on PKC (protein kinase C) activity. Enzyme activity was assayed by determining the incorporation of ^{32}P from [γ-^{32}P]ATP into calf thymus H1 histone (type III-S) at 30°C over a period of 3 min in the presence of 1 μM Ca^{2+}, 1 mM EGTA, and 100 μM phospholipid (phosphatidylcholine (PC)/phosphatidylserine (PS) (4:1 molar ratio) with various concentrations of inhalation anesthetics (halothane, enflurane, isoflurane). PKC was obtained from cerebral tissues of male Wistar/Slc rats and purified, using a previously described method [10]. Each of the examined inhalation anesthetics increased PKC activity in a dose-dependent manner.

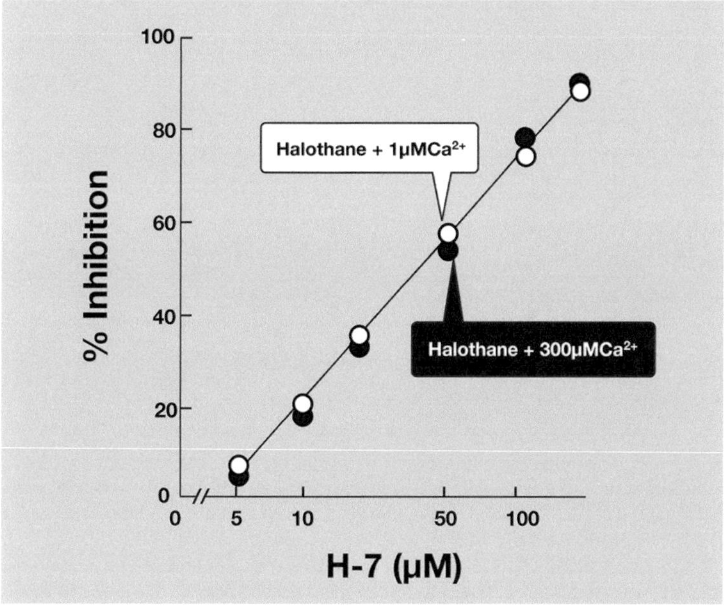

Figure 4. Effects of H-7, specific inhibitor of PKC, on halothane-activated PKC activity in the presence of low (1 μM) and high (0.3 mM) concentrations of Ca^{2+}. The concentration of halothane was 20 mM, whereas the other experimental conditions were the same as described in **Figure 3**. H-7 inhibited halothane-activated PKC activity in a dose-dependent manner.

3. Calming effect of local anesthetics on neutrophils

In contrast to general inhalation anesthetics, lidocaine has been found to inhibit protein kinase C in a manner competitive with phosphatidylserine as well as phosphorylation of the 47-kDa neutrophil cytoplasmic protein [11, 14, 15]. Thus, various stimulation-coupled responses of neutrophils, such as superoxide generation (**Figure 5**), depolarization of membrane potential (**Figure 6**), and transitional increase in intracellular Ca^{2+} (**Figure 7**), are suppressed by lidocaine. Other local anesthetics have also been shown to inhibit protein kinase C activity [15] and induce the same effects (**Figure 8**). These findings indicate that local anesthetics have unique calming effects on neutrophils as compared with inhalation anesthetics, which may reduce oxidative stress.

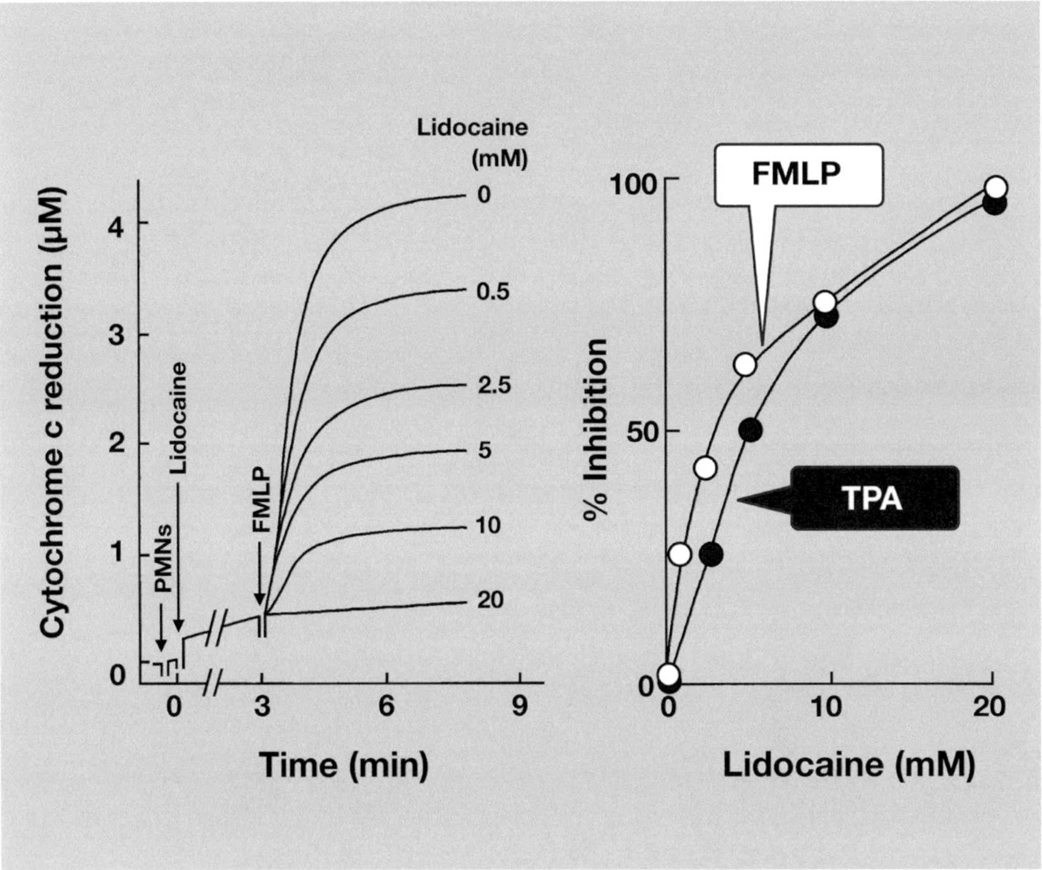

Figure 5. Effects of lidocaine on superoxide generation by neutrophils. Neutrophils were obtained from a guinea pig and suspended (1×10^6 cells·ml^{-1}) in KRP medium containing 10 mM glucose, 1.5 mM NaN_3, 1 mM Ca^{2+}, and 25 μM cytochrome c. After pre-incubation for 3 min at 37°C with various concentrations of lidocaine (0–20 mM), 100 nM FMLP (formyl-methionyl-leucyl-phenylalanine) or 0.5 nM TPA (12-O-tetradecanoylphorbol-13-acetate) was added. Superoxide generation by neutrophils was analyzed by determining the reduction of cytochrome c, which was measured at 550 nm with a reference wavelength of 540 nm. *Left panel*: Time course of cytochrome c reduction induced by FMLP-stimulated neutrophils. *Right panel*: Percent inhibition of reduction of cytochrome c in FMLP or TPA-stimulated neutrophils by lidocaine. These results indicated that lidocaine strongly inhibited superoxide generation in neutrophils stimulated by treatment with TPA or FMLP in a dose-dependent manner.

http://dx.doi.org/10.5772/66573

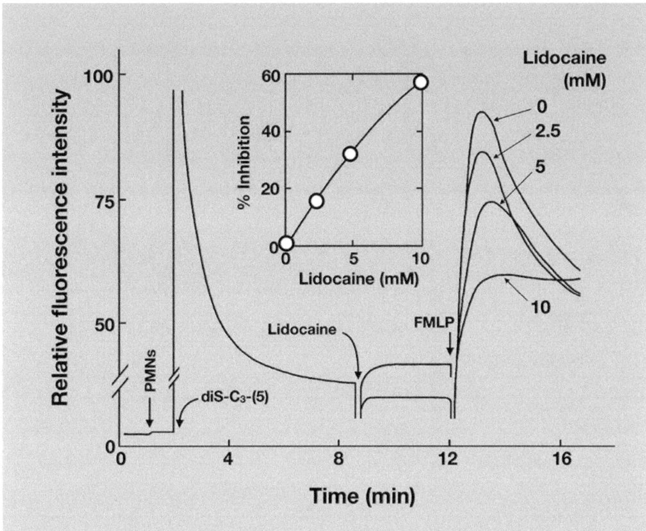

Figure 6. Effects of lidocaine on membrane potential in neutrophils. We used a cyanine dye method with diS-C3-(5). Neutrophils (1×10^6 cells·ml^{-1}) were obtained from a guinea pig and suspended in KRP medium containing 10 mM glucose, 1 mM Ca^{2+}, and 5 μM diS-C3-(5) at 37°C. After pre-incubation for 3 min with various concentrations of lidocaine, 100 nM FMLP was added. Changes in the fluorescence intensity of diS-C3-(5) were monitored at 670 nm after the dye had been exited at 622 nm. Downward deflections in the trace indicate uptake of diS-C3-(5) by the cells corresponding to hyperpolarization of the membrane potential. The inserted curved line graph indicates percent inhibition of fluorescence change by addition of lidocaine. Values were obtained by comparisons of peak values. These results indicated that lidocaine inhibited the membrane depolarization of neutrophils induced by FMLP, which was accompanied by superoxide generation.

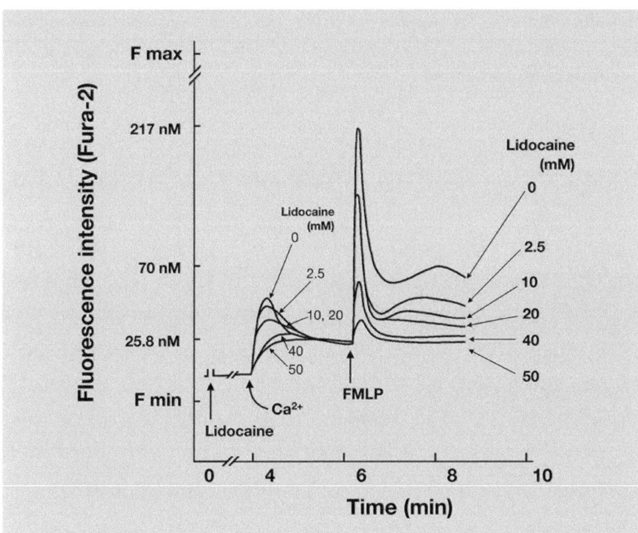

Figure 7. The effects of lidocaine on intracellular Ca^{2+} concentration. $[Ca^{2+}]_i$ in neutrophils was analyzed by determining the fluorescence intensity of Fura-2, a fluorescent indicator of intracellular calcium. Neutrophils were obtained from a guinea pig and suspended (1×10^6 cells·ml−^{1}) in Ca^{2+}-free KRP medium, then Fura-2 was added. Neutrophils were pre-incubated for 3 min with various concentrations of lidocaine at 37°C, then incubated with 1 mM Ca^{2+} for 2 min before addition of 50 nM FMLP. $[Ca^{2+}]_i$ was calculated based on the change in fluorescence intensity of Fura-2. A change in intensity indicated that lidocaine inhibited the increase in intracellular Ca^{2+} during the course of neutrophil activation.

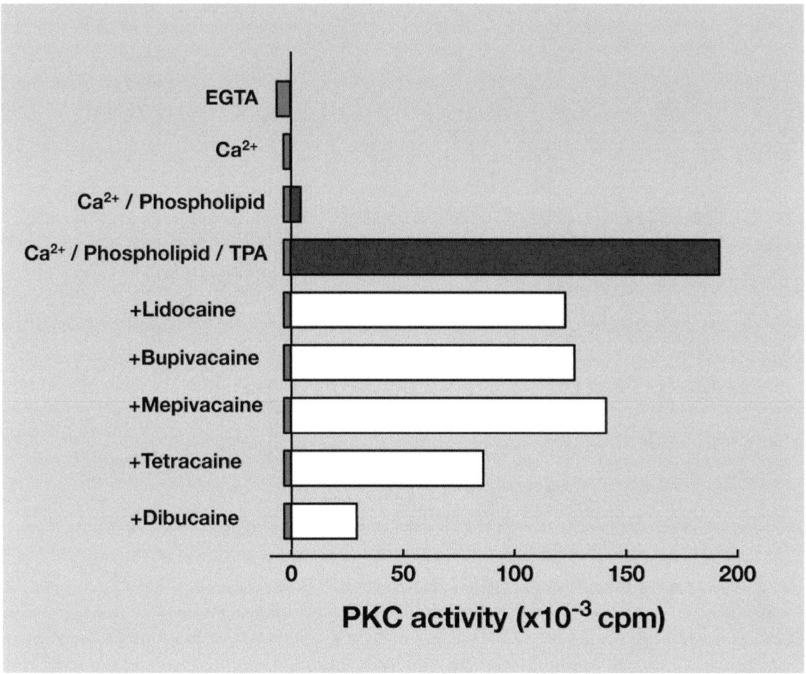

Figure 8. Effects of lidocaine and other local anesthetics on PKC activity in rat brain. PKC was obtained from a rat brain and purified using a method previously described [10]. Enzyme activity was assessed by measuring the incorporation of ^{32}P from [γ-^{32}P]ATP into H1 histone (type IIIs) at 30°C for 3 min. The medium contained 20 mM Tris-HCI (pH 7.5), 10 mM magnesium acetate, 0.2 mg·ml^{-1} histone, and 1 μM Ca^{2+}. The amounts of phospholipid (phosphatidylserine (PS)/ dipalmitoylphosphatidylcholine (DPPC), 1:4 molar ratio), TPA, and local anesthetics used were 100 μM, 100 nM and 0.5 mM, respectively. These results indicated that lidocaine and other local anesthetics inhibited PKC activity, with dibucaine shown to be the most potent inhibitor.

4. Novel method for determining antioxidant activity of medical agents

We developed a phycoerythrin fluorescence-based assay to determine the antioxidant activity of various medical agents including local anesthetics [3, 16, 17]. This assay system consists of B-phycoerythrin (B-PE) as a fluorescence molecule to show oxidative stress and 2,2′-azobis (2-amidinopropane) dihydrochloride (AAPH) as a hydrophilic oxidative stress simulator, which continuously generates peroxyl radicals at a constant rate, making it possible to easily evaluate the antioxidant activities of various medical agents [18]. Since the system is based on protein oxidation by peroxyl radicals, it is considered to be a model of in vivo ROS reactions. The detailed reactions of B-PE with AAPH can be illustrated as follows.

$$R-N=N-R \rightarrow R\bullet + N_2 + \bullet R \rightarrow (1-e)\,R-R \tag{1}$$

$$\searrow 2eR\bullet \tag{2}$$

$$R\bullet + O_2 \rightarrow RO_2\bullet \tag{3}$$

$$RO_2\bullet + B-PE \rightarrow \text{stable products} \tag{4}$$

$$RO_2 \bullet \; + A \rightarrow \text{stable products} \tag{5}$$

The structure of AAPH [HCl•NH=C(NH_2)-C(CH_3)$_2$-N=N-C(CH_3)$_2$-C(NH_2)=NH•HCl] is represented by "R-N=N-R", where "e" represents the efficiency of free radical generation and "A" is an antioxidant. AAPH undergoes thermal decomposition to yield free radicals (reaction (2)), which rapidly react with oxygen molecules nearby to produce peroxyl radicals (reaction (3)). With this assay, peroxyl radicals may attack B-PE, resulting in fluorescence decay (reaction (4)), which, if successful, may be scavenged by an antioxidant (reaction (5)).

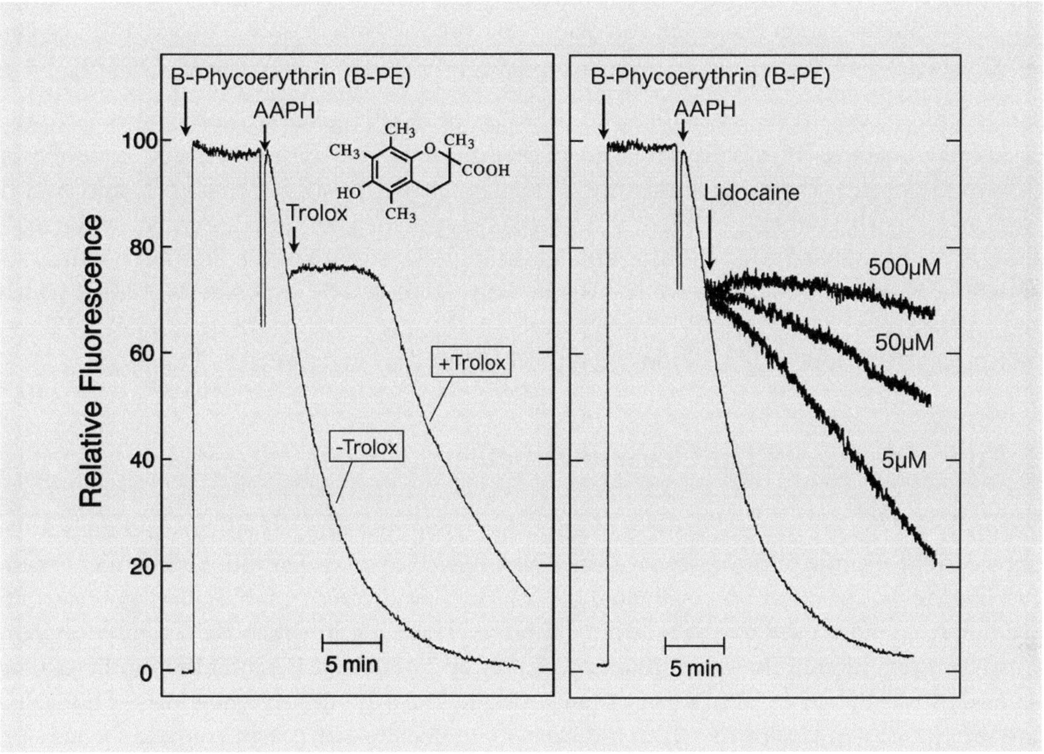

Figure 9. *Left panel*: Typical decay of fluorescence of B-PE (B-phycoerythrin) with AAPH (2,2′-azobis (2-amidinopropane) dihydrochloride) in Tris-HCl buffer (pH 7.4) at 38°C in the absence and presence of Trolox. The amounts of B-PE, AAPH, Trolox, and Tris-HCl buffer used were 1.78 nM, 6.25 mM, 4 μM, and 40 mM, respectively. The fluorescence excitation and emission wavelength were 545 nm (3-nm slit) and 575 nm (5-nm slit), respectively. Exposure of B-PE to peroxyl radicals generated by AAPH led to a decrease in B-PE fluorescence. This peroxidation process was efficiently inhibited by addition of Trolox, which has potent antioxidant activity. The characteristic features of this assay offer great advantages for determining the possible antioxidant activity of various compounds when added to the reaction mixture. *Right panel*: Effects of lidocaine on B-PE fluorescence decay. Although lidocaine did not completely abrogate the fluorescence decay of B-PE, it reduced the rate of decay in a dose-dependent manner. This finding indicated that lidocaine has an antioxidant function, though its potency is not as strong as that of Trolox.

The rate of peroxyl radical generation, R, from AAPH at a constant temperature is shown by Eq. (6) [19]:

$$R = K \times [AAPH] \tag{6}$$

where K is the rate constant for radical generation from AAPH and [AAPH] is the concentration of AAPH in M. The rate of radical generation is virtually constant during the first few hours of this assay [20], since the half-life of AAPH is approximately 175 h in neutral pH water at 37°C [19]. The rate of peroxyl radical generation at 38°C under the present assay conditions was $1.56 \times 10^{-6} \times [AAPH]$ ($M \cdot s^{-1}$) [3].

B-PE is a multisubunit protein extracted from the unicellular red alga, *Porphyridium cruentum* [16, 20]. Since it is easily oxidized, which decreases its fluorescence, B-PE functions as a reporting molecule of oxidative stress induced by peroxyl radicals from AAPH. In addition, because of its very high extinction coefficient and fluorescence quantum yields, B-PE can be readily detected by fluorescence spectroscopy at concentrations as low as 10^{-12} M [20].

For this assay, the fluorescence decay of B-PE by the AAPH-generated peroxyl radical was spectrophotometrically monitored at an excitation of 545 nm (3-nm slit) and emission of 575 nm (5-nm slit). The reaction mixture (2 ml) contained 1.78 nM B-PE and 6.25 mM AAPH in 40 mM Tris-HCl buffer (pH 7.4) at 38°C. Since the system is not closed, oxygen for the reactions is freely supplied from the atmosphere through the surface of the reaction mixture. As shown in **Figure 9**, B-PE fluorescence was linearly decreased by exposure to AAPH, which has a linear relationship with B-PE concentration. This peroxidative destruction of B-PE can be temporarily stopped by addition of a typical radical scavenger, such as Trolox.

5. Antioxidant activity of local anesthetics

We analyzed the antioxidant activity of lidocaine using this analysis system and the results showed that the rate of fluorescence decay was slowed in a concentration-dependent manner (**Figure 9**). The effect was evaluated by determining the percent inhibition against B-PE oxidation, an index used for the reactivity of peroxyl radicals, in which 100% inhibition indicates the same level of fluorescence decay as that by Trolox and 0% inhibition indicates the same decay as that in the absence of the antioxidant. The dose-dependent effects of lidocaine are summarized in **Figure 10**, which indicates that lidocaine has potent antioxidant activity, while other local anesthetics such as mepivacaine showed similar but slightly weaker effects.

Combined with the findings of neutrophils, local anesthetics have effects to counter oxidative stress in a manner opposite of inhalation anesthetics, indicating that use of local anesthetics can reverse the deleterious effects of inhalation anesthetics. Thus, from the standpoint of oxidative stress management, anesthesia with a combination of local and general inhalation anesthetics provides better anesthesia management. The advantage of local anesthetics in oxidative stress management was also revealed in a study by Budic et al., who examined cases of pediatric extremity surgery using pneumatic tourniquets [21]. They measured generation of the oxidative products malondialdehyde and protein carbonyl groups in plasma and found that peripheral nerve block anesthesia did not increase the levels after tourniquet release as compared with general anesthesia with sevoflurane, which significantly increased those levels. These findings indicate that regional anesthesia provides an antioxidant defense that is superior to that of general inhalation anesthesia.

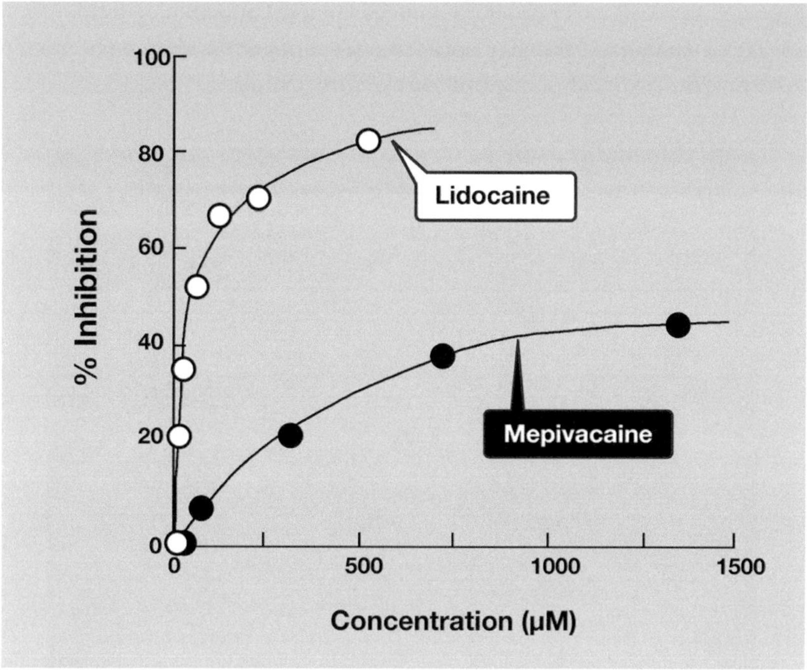

Figure 10. Dose-dependent effects of lidocaine and mepivacaine on B-PE fluorescence decay in the antioxidant assay system shown in **Figure 9**. These results indicated that both local anesthetics have a potent antioxidant activity.

6. Better intraoperative hemodynamic control by regional anesthesia

Regional anesthesia combined with general anesthesia provides not only better postoperative analgesia, but may also result in better intraoperative hemodynamic control than general anesthesia alone [22]. We demonstrated this advantage of regional anesthesia in an investigation of high-risk patients with severe cardiovascular disease classified as American Society of Anesthesiologists (ASA) physical status 3.

Patients undergoing elective open abdominal surgery were randomized into those receiving general anesthesia and a bilateral transversus abdominis plane block (TAPB) (Group T, $n = 33$), and those receiving general anesthesia alone (Group G, $n = 35$). The bilateral TAPB was performed after anesthesia induction using 40 ml of 0.3% ropivacaine, as shown in **Figure 11**. We compared the groups for intraoperative hemodynamic stability, anesthesia emergence time, amounts of anesthetics and opioids given, and frequency of emergency treatment with a cardiovascular agent. A hemodynamically stable period was defined as the time when systolic blood pressure and heart rate were 70–110% of their preanesthesia value. The ratio of hemodynamically stable time to total operative time was used as an index of hemodynamic stability.

Hemodynamically stable time was greater in Group T than Group G (**Figure 12**), while sevoflurane concentration, amount of fentanyl given, and frequency of vasopressor use were lower, and anesthesia emergence time was shorter in the Group T patients (**Figure 13**). These findings indicate that the combination of TAPB with general anesthesia promotes intraoperative hemodynamic stability and early emergence from general anesthesia, while it also provides good postoperative analgesia. Furthermore, the advantageous effects obtained with TAPB may also be seen with use of other regional anesthetic protocols.

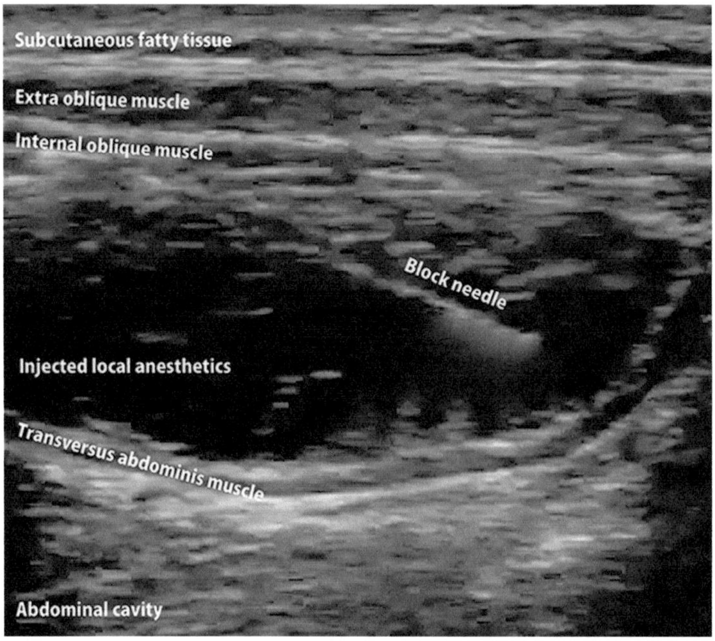

Figure 11. Ultrasound image of abdominal wall during transversus abdominis plane block (TAPB).

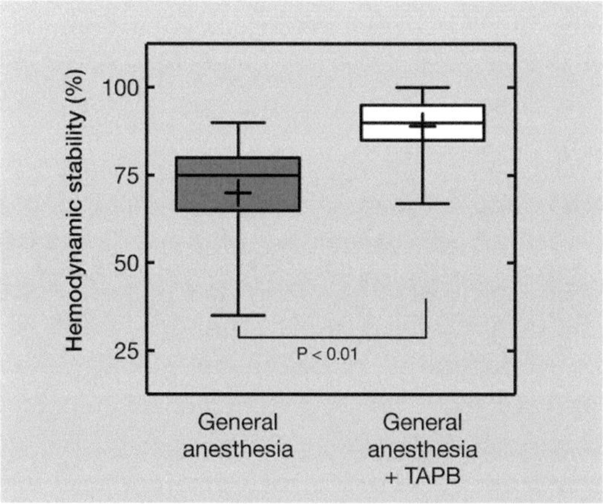

Figure 12. Box-plot for comparison of intraoperative hemodynamic stability between Group G (general anesthesia alone, $n = 35$) and Group T (general anesthesia plus TAPB, $n = 33$). The period during the operation when both systolic blood pressure and heart rate were within 70–110% of their pre-anesthesia value was defined as the hemodynamic stable time. The ratio of hemodynamic stable time to total operative time was used as an indicator of hemodynamic stability. The stability ratio was significantly higher in Group T (91%, range 50–100%) than in Group G (79, 40–91%), indicating greater hemodynamic stability in Group T. Values are presented as the median and minimum-maximum range.

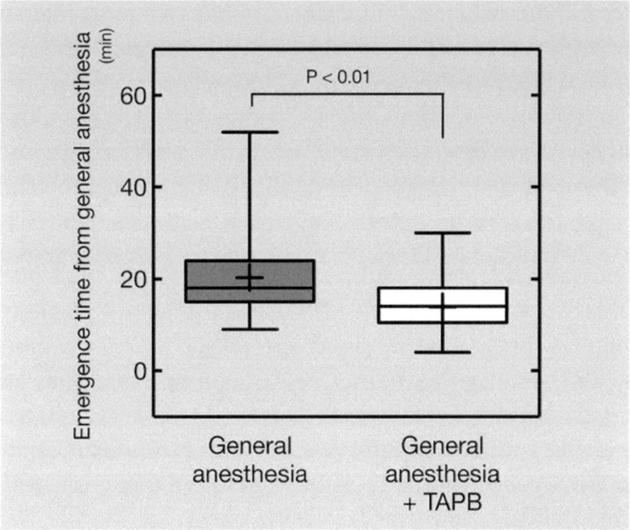

Figure 13. Box-plot for comparison of anesthesia emergence time between Group G (general anesthesia alone, $n = 35$) and Group T (general anesthesia plus TAPB, $n = 33$). Anesthesia emergence time was defined as the time from completion of surgery to extubation. That time was significantly shorter in Group T (14 min, range 4–30 min) than in Group G (18 min, 9–52 min). Values are presented as the median and minimum-maximum range.

It is important for anesthesiologists to offer effective anesthesia management for high-risk patients with severe cardiovascular disease [23], as they frequently require special treatment with a variety of expensive drugs and increased medical staffing. This combined regional and general anesthesia technique is si mple and easy to perform, and its advantages include relief of the burden to the anesthesiologist and reduced medical costs for such high-risk cases, as well as improved patient safety.

7. Interim summary

Combined use of regional with general anesthesia is advantageous to decrease oxidative stress and also provides better intraoperative hemodynamics than general anesthesia alone. Namely, it compensates for the shortcomings of inhalation anesthetics and improves anesthesia management quality. Importantly, the hemodynamic stabilizing effects of regional anesthesia in high-risk patients provide a great advantage for the anesthesiologist to perform anesthesia management, even when additional efforts to perform regional anesthesia are required.

8. Addition of low-molecular weight dextran to local anesthetics: enhancement of analgesic effect and reduction of toxicity

Regional anesthesia, though useful, has some limitations. It is often performed as a single-shot procedure with a large dose of a local anesthetic drug, except for cases of epidural anesthesia, which is usually performed with insertion of a catheter for continuous administration. Therefore, prolonging analgesia without toxicity is clinically important for most regional anesthesia procedures. Furthermore, when performed in combination with general anesthesia, a prolonged analgesia duration is required, because the period of postoperative analgesia is shortened depending on operation time. In light of these limitations and demands, studies aimed at improving the effects of local anesthetics have been performed, some of which have provided evidence showing that addition of low-molecular weight dextran (LMWD) to a local anesthetic and epinephrine mixture when given as infiltration anesthesia [24], or to a local anesthetic alone when performing a regional block [25] safely prolonged the effective action by reducing systemic absorption.

We demonstrated this favorable effect of LMWD as an adjuvant in patients being prepared for laparoscopic colon surgery, who received anesthesia with a combination of TAPB and rectus sheath block (RSB) using either 80 ml of 0.2% levobupivacaine in saline (control group, $n = 27$) or 80 ml of 0.2% levobupivacaine in 8% LMWD (LMWD group, $n = 27$). Following anesthesia induction, the combined block was performed under a double-blind condition. Levobupivacaine plasma concentration and postoperative analgesia were assessed using a numerical rating scale (NRS).

In the LMWD group, the time to reach the maximum plasma concentration of levobupivacaine (T_{max}) was longer (73 ± 25 vs. 51 ± 30 min, $P = 0.006$) and the maximum plasma concentration (C_{max}) was lower (1141 ± 287 vs. 1410 ± 322 ng·ml^{-1}, $P = 0.004$), as compared to the control group (**Figure 14**). The area under the plasma concentration-time curve (AUC) from 0 to

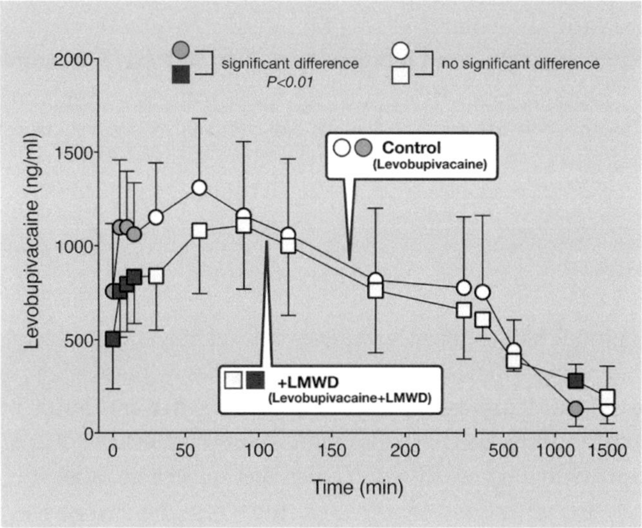

Figure 14. Changes in plasma concentration of levobupivacaine in patients receiving levobupivacaine at 160 mg (0.2%) in saline (control group, $n = 27$) or an 8% low-molecular weight dextran solution (LMWD group, $n = 27$) following a bilateral transversus abdominis block (TAPB) or rectus sheath block (RSB). Error bars show the SD and time 0 indicates completion of the nerve block procedure. In the control group, the plasma concentration of levobupivacaine quickly rose just after performing the nerve block. In the LMWD group, that rose in a more gradual manner with a lower maximum concentration. Subsequently, the plasma concentration of levobupivacaine gradually decreased in both groups, though a faster decline was seen in the control group. At 1200 min after performing the block, the plasma concentration of levobupivacaine was significantly higher in the LMWD group as compared to the control group.

240 min was also lower (172,484 ± 50,502 vs. 229,124 ± 87,254 ng min·ml^{-1}, $P = 0.007$) in the LMWD group, while their NRS scores up to 24 h after surgery were reduced (**Figure 15**). Also, rescue treatment with IV flurbiprofen (50 mg) was utilized significantly less often in the LMWD group. No typical adverse effects, such as wound infection, delayed wound healing, tissue necrosis, or prolonged abnormal sensory disorder over the area of injection, were observed in either group. The lower C_{max} value was associated with reduced risk of levobupivacaine toxicity, while lower AUC indicated that the addition of LMWD reduced systemic absorption of levobupivacaine. Thus, those results indicated that addition of LMWD enhances analgesia for a longer duration along with decreased risk of local anesthetic toxicity.

However, the efficacy of dextrans including LMWD remains controversial, as several subsequent studies have reported an absence of any substantial difference in analgesic duration with their addition [26, 27]. These inconsistent findings related to the effects of dextrans may be due to differences in regional anesthesia techniques. Recent advances in ultrasound technology have greatly increased the accuracy of various types of nerve blocks, thus local anesthetics can be precisely injected into the target compartment or very near the target without complications in this modern era. Such improved accuracy may reveal the effects of dextrans not seen with classical techniques.

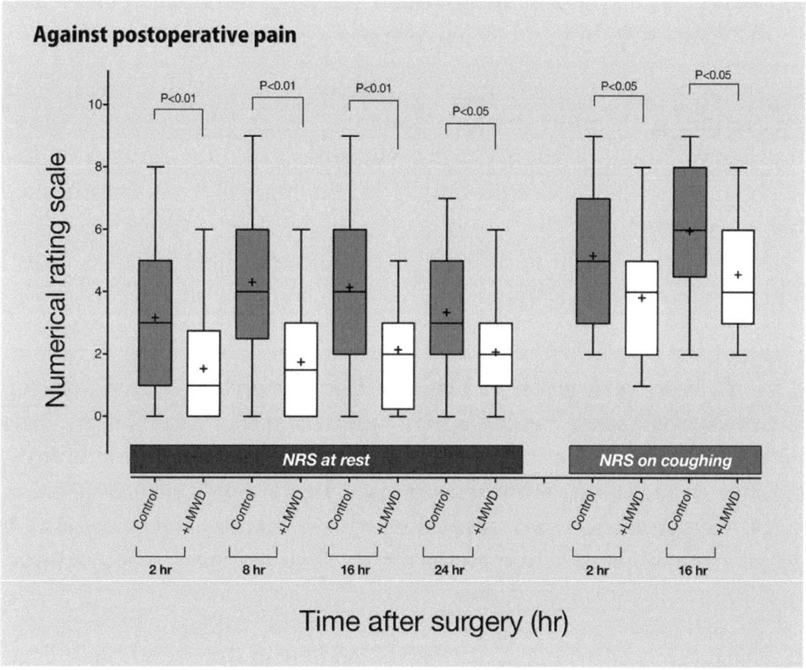

Figure 15. Box-plots for comparing postoperative pain between the control and LMWD groups at rest and during coughing using a numerical rating scale (NRS). Details of the nerve block procedures used in each group are described in the legend to **Figure 14**. NRS scores at both rest and during coughing at all time points up to 24 h after surgery were significantly lower in the LMWD group as compared to the control group.

Nevertheless, use of LMWD as a local anesthetic adjuvant has nearly been forgotten in recent years. We rediscovered its value with the aid of ultrasound technology and found that use of LMWD with a local anesthetic mixture is a good option to further improve the performance of TAPB or RSB, and likely other regional anesthesia procedures as well. Extension of the analgesia period to the next day after surgery by a simple single-shot approach is fully adequate for most surgery patients, making unnecessary the complicated procedure of inserting a catheter for continuous administration and subsequent management during the postoperative period. Thus, use of LMWD makes regional anesthesia more easily accessible to many anesthesiologists and may open a new horizon for them.

9. Novel clinical application of older mature nerve block technique by use of ultrasound technology: caudal block

Improvements in ultrasound technology have resulted in the return of some older mature nerve block techniques to clinical importance, as also seen with LMWD. One of those is caudal block. Since a high level of skill is required to safely perform an adequate caudal block in older adults, because of anatomical deformity of the sacrum associated with aging, it is rarely performed in elderly patients and generally believed to be a special nerve block technique for use in pediatric cases. However, ultrasound technology has made it much easier to safely perform a caudal block with high consistency in older patients [2].

We studied the clinical usefulness and availability of a caudal block for urinary catheter-induced bladder discomfort in adult patients, which is common in those who have undergone urinary catheterization during surgery. In some cases, the discomfort is severe, causing restlessness and agitation after emergence from anesthesia, with postoperative recovery sometimes disrupted due to the continual uneasiness. These adverse effects are more pronounced in middle-aged and elderly male patients due to anatomic considerations.

Muscarinic receptor antagonists, such as ketamine and gabapentin, have been shown to be effective for relieving postoperative bladder discomfort caused by a catheter. However, they may alter hemodynamics, leading to dry mouth or excessive sedation. In view of such unwanted side effects, these agents may not be best for treatment of bladder discomfort in all patients. Since caudal block anesthesia is used in the fields of urological and gynecological surgery, we speculated that ultrasound-guided single shot anesthesia by a caudal block would be a reliable and safe method for relief of urinary catheter-induced bladder discomfort.

We enrolled male patients (ASA I-II) older than 50 years who were scheduled for cervical spine surgery, and allocated them to either the caudal block (Group CB, $n = 22$) or non-block (Group NB, $n = 22$) group. Following induction of anesthesia, urinary catheterization was performed using a 16-F Foley catheter. In Group CB, an ultrasound-guided single shot caudal block was additionally performed before the start of surgery using an 8-ml mixture of 0.3% ropivacaine and 100 μg of fentanyl. Group NB did not undergo a caudal block or receive any other drugs. Thereafter, spine surgery started. The severity of urinary catheter-related discomfort was assessed at 0 (just after arrival in the post-anesthesia care unit), then 2, 10, and 18 h after the operation.

Following are details of our method for ultrasound-guided caudal block. With the patient in a prone position, the location and structure of the sacral hiatus are confirmed on sonographic transverse and longitudinal images. Next, a 23-gauge block needle is inserted in the direction of the sacral canal through the sacral hiatus while monitoring real-time sonographic images (**Figure 16**), then the tip of the block needle is inserted into the sacral canal at least 1 cm ahead. After negative aspiration, a mixture of ropivacaine and fentanyl is injected. Injection of that mixture into epidural space is confirmed by ultrasound images showing that the block needle is properly inserted in the direction of the sacral canal through the sacral hiatus, while a small fraction of injection fluid in the depth of the sacral canal shows reverse spreading into the canal opening portion near the sacral hiatus.

All caudal block procedures in this study were guided by ultrasound and successfully performed without severe difficulties. Following surgery, the incidence rate of urinary catheter-induced discomfort was significantly reduced in Group CB as compared to Group NB (**Figure 17**). There were no complications related to caudal block anesthesia, including bleeding or hematoma at the injection site. No motor block of the extremities was observed and none of the patients required re-catheterization due to urinary retention after catheter removal. These results showed that ultrasound-guided single shot caudal block anesthesia can reduce the incidence and severity of postoperative urinary catheter-induced bladder discomfort.

Our findings of reduced difficulties and improved reliability with use of ultrasound guidance indicate that a caudal block can be used in adults for bladder discomfort treatment, as well as various other procedures performed in the lower abdomen region, including pelvic, bladder, perineal, genital, rectal, and anal surgery, namely, inguinal and femoral herniorrhaphy, cystoscopy, urethral surgery, prostatectomy, hemorrhoidectomy, vaginal hysterectomy, and other surgeries of the perineum, anus, and rectum. The effectiveness of a caudal block for postoperative analgesia in patients undergoing such operations is also promising.

We now consider that a caudal block can be accurately and safely performed in adults with ultrasound guidance. In addition, its application in combination with general anesthesia is expected to improve the quality of anesthesia, as shown with TAPB. In particular, a caudal block may be more suitable for high-risk cases, as the technique is simple with minimum hemodynamic effects.

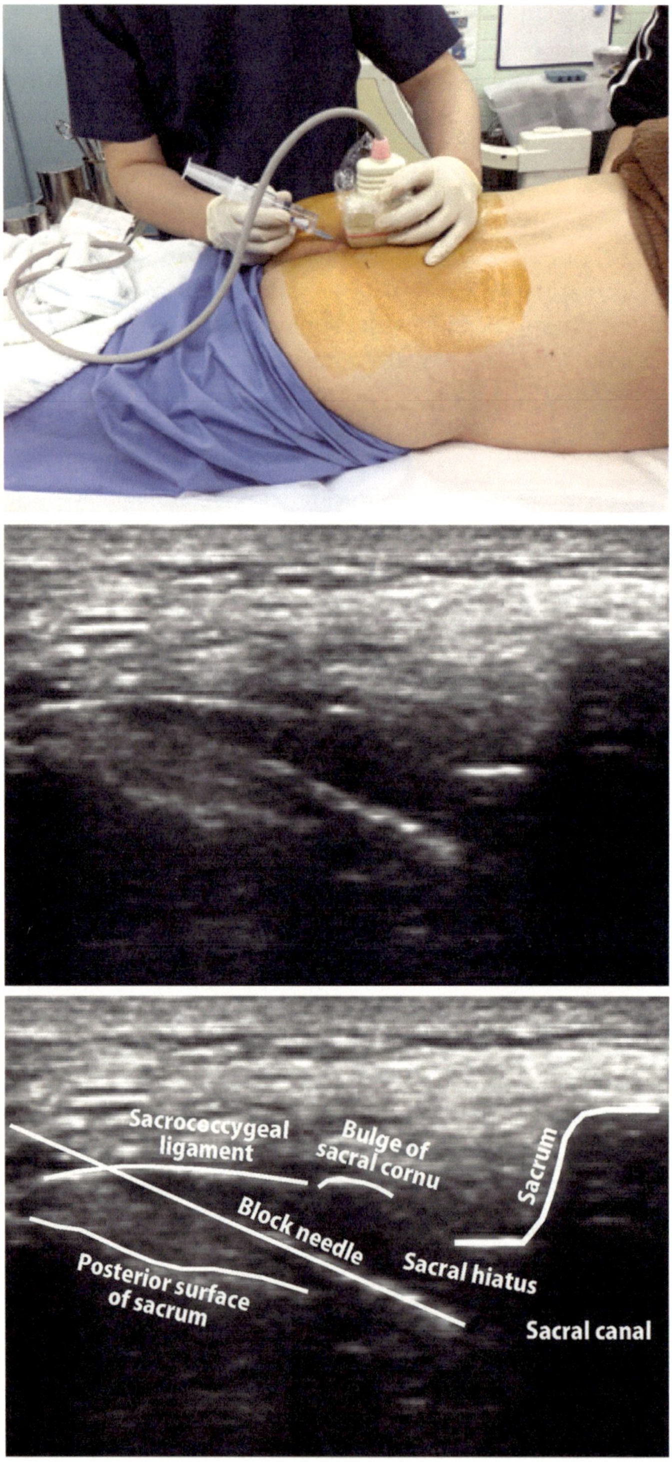

Figure 16. Ultrasound probe positioning and ultrasound images obtained during performance of caudal block.

http://dx.doi.org/10.5772/66573

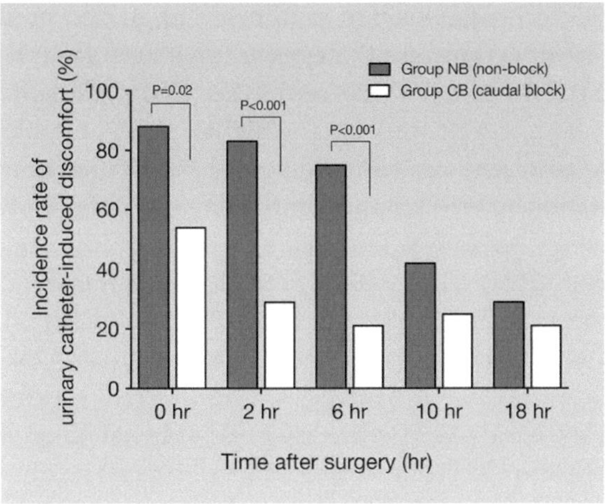

Figure 17. Effects of caudal block to alleviate catheter-induced bladder discomfort. The patients in Group CB ($n = 22$) received a caudal block with 8 ml of 0.3% ropivacaine and 100 μg of fentanyl after anesthesia induction, while those in Group NB ($n = 22$) did not receive a caudal block. The incidence rate of urinary catheter-induced bladder discomfort was significantly lower in Group CB when compared to Group NB at 0, 2, and 6 h after surgery.

10. Importance of optimal in-line positioning of ultrasound image monitor for accurate and quick nerve block

Although ultrasound guidance for providing regional anesthesia has great potential, as described above, it is not easy to perform for novice practitioners. When using ultrasound, the operator is required to mentally restructure two-dimensional images presented on a display into the three-dimensional relationship of the target with the needle. This spatial conversion represents a major hurdle for precise performance of an ultrasound-guided procedure. It has been shown that an ergonomic layout of the equipment utilized with the patient that allows the operator's gaze to run in a straight line from the puncture site to the ultrasound image display along the direction of needle insertion is important for accurate and quick spatial recognition of the needle position [28]. However, since the operating room can become crowded with numerous medical devices, the ultrasound machine is sometimes positioned out of the line of sight of the puncture field, which disturbs spatial recognition of the needle position for the operator, increasing the difficulty of the procedure. Based on these considerations, we speculated that the position of the ultrasound image display in relation to the operator is a vital factor for achieving success with ultrasound-guided procedures.

Imaging technology has progressed significantly in recent years and modern devices are widely used in the medical field. In particular, digital tablets, such as the iPad and iPad Mini (Apple Japan LLC, Tokyo, Japan), are gaining use as viewers for X-ray and 3-dimensional images during surgical procedures. These small lightweight displays can be easily placed in nearly any position by the operator and may be ideal for use during ultrasound-guided procedures.

To verify the importance of image position in ultrasound guided procedures, we developed a system for wireless real-time transfer of images vfrom an ultrasound image display consisting of a wireless video transmitter (VT-100; Scalar Co., Tokyo, Japan) and an iPad Mini. The VT-100, a battery-operated, ultra-compact, and lightweight portable transmitter (approximately 290 g, including batteries) can simultaneously send video images from a single iPad Mini to other multiple iPads by Wi-Fi with a short delay of 0.067 s. However, the resolution of transferred images is somewhat low at 320 × 240 dots per inch (dpi), with a frame rate of more than 15 frames per second (fps). Thus, we have made fine adjustments to the image quality to allow the VT-100 to be suitable for ultrasound image transmission. The modified VT-100 is connected to an ultrasound machine (ProSound Alpha 7; Hitachi-Aloka Medical Ltd., Tokyo, Japan) via a video cable and ultrasound images are transferred to a single iPad Mini via Wi-Fi (**Figure 18**). Dedicated software (AirMicro; Scalar Co.) is installed on the iPad Mini for viewing images. Furthermore, the iPad Mini is attached to a special flexible arm with a holder for easy positioning in the area around the operating table.

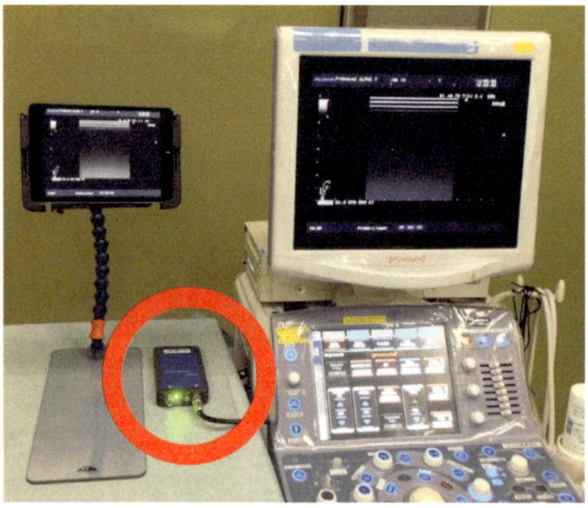

Figure 18. iPad Mini (Apple Japan LLC, Tokyo, Japan), VT-100 wireless video transmitter encircled in red (Scalar Co., Tokyo, Japan), and ProSound Alpha 7 ultrasound equipment (Hitachi-Aloka Medical Ltd., Tokyo, Japan). With our method, ultrasound image signals from the ProSound Alpha 7 are transmitted by a conventional coaxial video cable to the VT-100, then sent wirelessly to the iPad Mini by Wi-Fi without any image reproduction delay.

We investigated success rate and time required for ultrasound-guided radial artery catheterization performed by novice residents when using this system in two image positions (**Figure 19**). The operators were asked to insert a catheter into the radial artery using a short-axis out-of-plane approach with a crossover method (**Figure 20**) with use of either the ultrasound machine placed at the head side of the patient across the targeted forearm (conventional method, $n = 20$) or the iPad ultrasound imaging transmission system (iPad Mini + VT-100 method, $n = 20$). When the latter was employed, the iPad was positioned so that the ultrasound images were viewed above the forearm in alignment with the operator's eyes and direction of needle puncture.

http://dx.doi.org/10.5772/66573

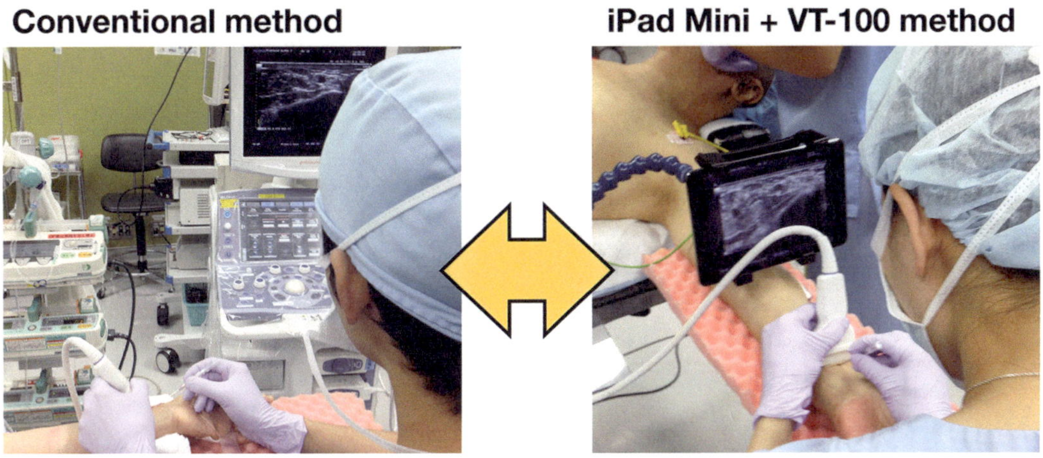

Figure 19. Positional relationships with conventional method and iPad Mini with VT100 method. With the conventional method, the ultrasound machine (ProSound Alpha 7) is placed at the head side of the patient and the puncture operator stands on the caudal side, with the patient forearm between them. With the iPad Mini with VT100 method, the axis running from the eye of the operator to the puncture needle and ultrasound image displayed on the iPad Mini are aligned as closely as possible along a straight line.

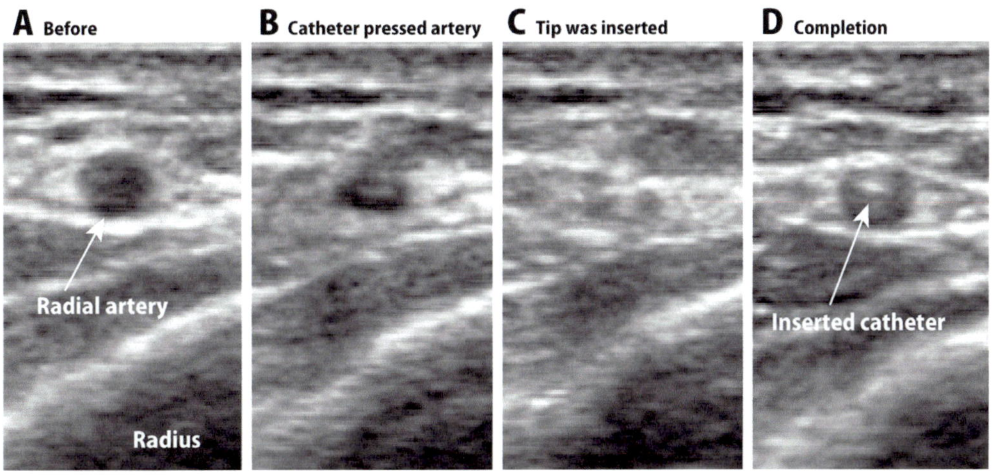

Figure 20. Representative series of four ultrasound images obtained during insertion of a radial artery catheter. A:before catheter insersion, B and C :during catheter insertion, D:completion of catheter insertion

We found that the success rate was significantly higher (100 vs. 70%, $p < 0.02$) and catheterization time significantly shorter (28.5 ± 7.5 vs. 68.2 ± 14.3 s, $p < 0.001$) with the iPad system (iPad Mini + VT-100 method) as compared to the ultrasound machine alone (conventional method). These results indicated that alignment of the visual axis of the operator, ultrasound images, and direction of needle puncture increased success rate and also reduced procedure time when performing ultrasound-guided catheterization (**Figure 21**).

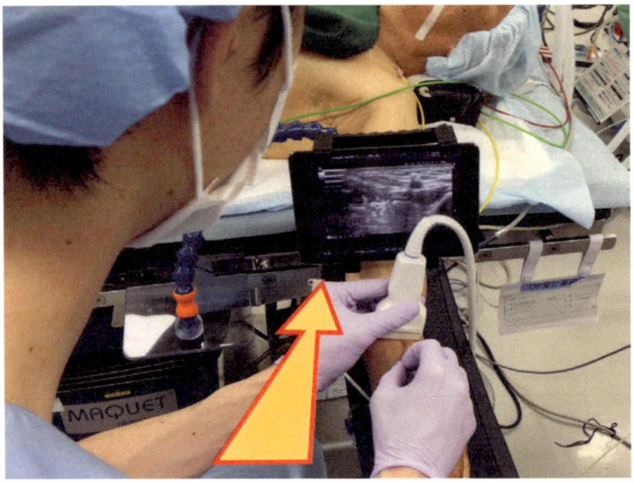

Figure 21. An ergonomic in-line arrangement of the image display, direction of needle insertion, and visual axis of the operator is crucial for successful and quick completion of ultrasound-guided procedures.

The position of the ultrasound image display is sometimes overlooked. However, we have found it to be a key point for successful and easy completion of ultrasound-guided procedures, especially when performed by practitioners with a low level of experience. For this purpose, our iPad system may be effective. In addition, it allows the ultrasound machine to be placed behind the operator, with only the display in front of their face, thus enabling a nerve block to be performed with overhand movements (**Figure 22**).

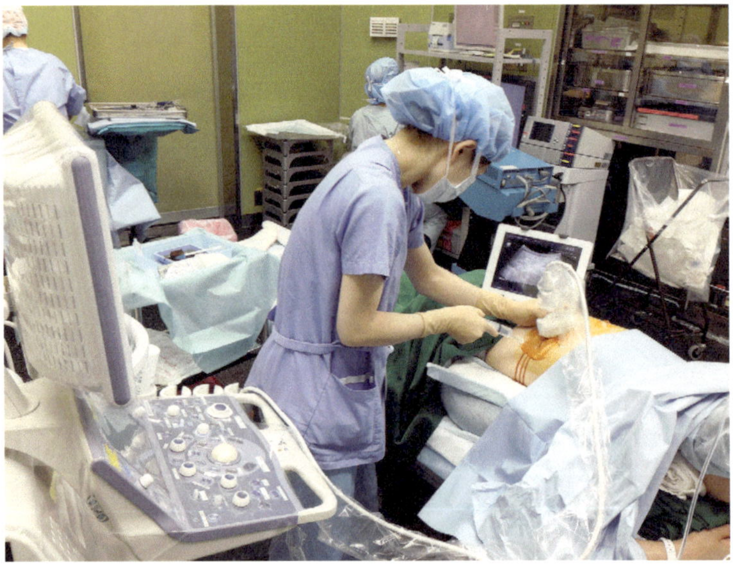

Figure 22. As shown in this representative image, the ultrasound machine is positioned behind the operator, who performs a paravertebral nerve block procedure on a prone patient while observing ultrasound images on an iPad.

11. Points of concern and disadvantages associated with performing regional anesthesia with general anesthesia

When using epidural anesthesia in combination with general anesthesia, it is highly recommended to insert the epidural catheter and then inject a test dose of the local anesthetic solution prior to the anesthesia induction, as this sequence allows for early recognition of severe complications, such as intrathecal or intravascular injection of the local anesthetic agent, or nerve injury caused by the epidural needle. In other recent cases when regional anesthesia was used, some anesthesiologists employed an ultrasound technique following anesthesia induction. With ultrasound imaging, the positions of the block needle, nerves, and blood vessels, as well as spread of the local anesthetic solution when performing regional anesthesia are clearly and accurately shown, thus ensuring the safety of the procedure even under an anesthetized condition in which the patient is unconscious. Nevertheless, there is no doubt that accidental nerve injury, as well as intravascular or unintended injection of the local anesthetic solution remain major threats for safety in all cases, which must be noted when performing regional anesthesia.

In a review conducted by the Japanese Society of Anesthesiologists of cases treated at certified training hospitals in Japan between 1999 and 2001, a higher incidence of intraoperative coronary ischemia was found in laparotomy patients anesthetized by inhalation general anesthesia in combination with regional anesthesia as compared to those who received general anesthesia alone [29]. Those findings indicated the possibility that a combined regional and general anesthesia technique might be unsuitable for patients with severe coronary diseases. On the other hand, TAPB and RSB techniques for a laparotomy have only been widely utilized in the most recent decade, thus it is reasonable to assume that cases of regional anesthesia included in that report were mainly epidural anesthesia. The combination of epidural anesthesia with general anesthesia can sometimes induce severe hypotension, which might have induced coronary ischemia in those patients. Furthermore, hypotensive effects might be more critical in patients with low output syndrome. However, as shown in our study of general anesthesia with TAPB, a peripheral nerve block does not usually induce hypotension, because it has a limited effect on the sympathetic nervous system as compared with epidural anesthesia. Thus, as long as an appropriate regional anesthesia method is carefully chosen, combined regional and general anesthesia should not be contraindicated in patients with severe coronary disease or low ejection fraction, though special caution is required for management of such high-risk patients.

12. Conclusion

Use of regional anesthesia in combination with general anesthesia provides important advantages for management of oxidative stress as well as control of hemodynamics during surgery. For improving the performance of regional anesthesia, addition of LMWD as an adjuvant to the local anesthetic solution is quite effective. In addition, ultrasound technology is very helpful to make regional anesthesia easier and safer to perform, while it is also valuable for reevaluation of caudal block treatment in adults. Utilization of a caudal block technique along with ultrasound guidance may be effective for adult patients undergoing surgery in the lower abdomen region, especially high-risk cases, as the technique is simple with minimum hemodynamic effects. We have also found that placement of ultrasound images in a proper in-line position by use of an iPad and the VT-100 image transfer system helps to facilitate accurate and quick needle insertion to the target, especially for novice practitioners. When considering these advantages of regional anesthesia and its advancement with the help of ultrasound technology, it is expected that the combined use of regional and general anesthesia will become more common for anesthetic management in the near future. Even though additional time is needed, regional anesthesia in conjunction with general anesthesia should be considered in all cases

Author details

Masahiko Tsuchiya

Address all correspondence to: oxymasa@ea.mbn.or.jp; oxymasa@gmail.com

Department of Anesthesiology, Osaka City University Medical School, Osaka, Japan

References

[1] Tsuchiya M, Kyoh Y. Key points for intraoperative management of percutaneous endoscopic lumbar discectomy (PELD) for anesthesiologists. *Minerva Anestesiol* 2013; **79**: 1318–9.

[2] Tsuchiya M, Kyoh Y, Mizutani K, Yamashita J, Hamada T. Ultrasound-guided single shot caudal block anesthesia reduces postoperative urinary catheter-induced discomfort. *Minerva Anestesiol* 2013; **79**: 1381–8.

[3] Kang MY, Tsuchiya M, Packer L, Manabe M. In vitro study on antioxidant potential of various drugs used in the perioperative period. *Acta Anaesthesiol Scand* 1998; **42**: 4–12.

[4] Tsuchiya M, Asada A, Inoue M. Significance of reactive oxygen species in vivo. *Japan J Intens Care Med* 2003; **27**: 649–60.

[5] Tsuchiya M, Sato EF, Inoue M, Asada A. Open abdominal surgery increases intraoperative oxidative stress: can it be prevented? *Anesth Analg* 2008; **107**: 1946–52.

[6] Suehiro K, Tanaka K, Matsuura T, et al. Preoperative hydroperoxide concentrations are associated with a risk of postoperative complications after cardiac surgery. *Anaesth Intensive Care* 2014; **42**: 487–94.

[7] Tsuchiya M, Tomoda M, Ueda W, Hirakawa M. Halothane enhances the phosphorylation of H1 histone and rat brain cytoplasmic proteins by protein kinase C. *Life Sci* 1990; **46**: 819–25.

[8] Tsuchiya M, Tomoda M, Ueda W, Hirakawa M. Inhalational anesthetics activate protein kinase C. *Journal of Clinical and Experimental Medicine* 1989; **150**: 697–8.

[9] Tsuchiya M, Tomoda M, Ueda W, Hirakawa M. Effect of halothan on protein kinase C activity. *Anesthesia and Resuscitation* 1990; **26**: 219–26.

[10] Tsuchiya M, Okimasu E, Ueda W, Hirakawa M, Utsumi K. Halothane, an inhalation anesthetic, activates protein kinase C and superoxide generation by neutrophils. *FEBS Lett* 1988; **242**: 101–5.

[11] Tomoda MK, Tsuchiya M, Ueda W, Hirakawa M, Utsumi K. Lidocaine inhibits stimulation-coupled responses of neutrophils and protein kinase C activity. *Physiol Chem Phys Med NMR* 1990; **22**: 199–210.

[12] Tsuchiya M, Takahashi M, Tomoda M, Ueda W, Hirakawa M. Halothane impairs the bioenergetic functions of isolated rat liver mitochondria. *Toxicol Appl Pharmacol* 1990; **104**: 466–75.

[13] Kevin LG, Novalija E, Riess ML, Camara AK, Rhodes SS, Stowe DF. Sevoflurane exposure generates superoxide but leads to decreased superoxide during ischemia and reperfusion in isolated hearts. *Anesth Analg* 2003; **96**: 949–55.

[14] Tomoda M, Ueda W, Tsuchiya M, Hirakawa M. Effects of lidocaine on stimulation-coupled responses of neutrophils and protein kinase C activity. *Masui* 1992; **41**: 369–75.

[15] Tsuchiya M, Tomoda M, Ueda W, Hirakawa M. Local anesthetics inhibit protein kinase C and active oxygen generation in neutrophils. *Journal of Clinical and Experimental Medicine* 1989; **150**: 569–70.

[16] Tsuchiya M, Scita G, Freisleben HJ, Kagan VE, Packer L. Antioxidant radical-scavenging activity of carotenoids and retinoids compared to alpha-tocopherol. *Methods Enzymol* 1992; **213**: 460–72.

[17] Tsuchiya M, Kagan VE, Freisleben HJ, Manabe M, Packer L. Antioxidant activity of alpha-tocopherol, beta-carotene, and ubiquinol in membranes: cis-parinaric acid-incorporated liposomes. *Methods Enzymol* 1994; **234**: 371–83.

[18] Tsuchiya M, Kang MY, Tokai H, et al. New antioxidant assay system reveals potent antioxidant activity of calcium channel blockers and steroids. *Journal of the Japanese Society of Intensive Care Medicine* 1999; **6**: 103–7.

[19] Niki E. Free radical initiators as source of water- or lipid-soluble peroxyl radicals. *Methods Enzymol* 1990; **186**: 100–8.

[20] Glazer AN. Fluorescence-based assay for reactive oxygen species: a protective role for creatinine. *FASEB J* 1988; **2**: 2487–91.

[21] Budic I, Pavlovic D, Cvetkovic T, et al. The effects of different anesthesia techniques on free radical production after tourniquet-induced ischemia-reperfusion injury at children's age. *Vojnosanit Pregl* 2010; **67**: 659–64.

[22] Tsuchiya M, Takahashi R, Furukawa A, Suehiro K, Mizutani K, Nishikawa K. Transversus abdominis plane block in combination with general anesthesia provides better intra-operative hemodynamic control and quicker recovery than general anesthesia alone in high-risk abdominal surgery patients. *Minerva Anestesiol* 2012; **78**: 1241–7.

[23] Mizutani K, Suwa K, Tsuchiya M. Illustration of O2 and CO2 recirculation to interpret respiratory and circulatory physiology. *J Clin Anesth* 2015; **27**: 363–5.

[24] Ueda W, Hirakawa M, Mori K. Inhibition of epinephrine absorption by dextran. *Anesthesiology* 1985; **62**: 72–5.

[25] Hamada T, Tsuchiya M, Mizutani K, et al. Levobupivacaine-dextran mixture for transversus abdominis plane block and rectus sheath block in patients undergoing laparoscopic colectomy: a randomised controlled trial. *Anaesthesia* 2016; **71**: 411–6.

[26] Kingsnorth AN, Wijesinha SS, Grixti CJ. Evaluation of dextran with local anaesthesia for short-stay inguinal herniorraphy. *Ann R Coll Surg Engl* 1979; **61**: 456–8.

[27] Buckley FP, Fink BR. Duration of action of nerve blocks produced by mixtures of local anesthetics and low molecular weight dextran: studies in rat infraorbital nerve blocks. *Anesth Analg* 1981; **60**: 142–5.

[28] Tsuchiya M, Mizutani K, Funai Y, Nakamoto T. In-line positioning of ultrasound images using wireless remote display system with tablet computer facilitates ultrasound-guided radial artery catheterization. *J Clin Monit Comput* 2016; **30**: 101–6.

[29] Irita K, Kawashima Y, Morita K, et al. Life-threatening coronary ischemia in the operating room: analysis of annual survey from 1999 to 2001 conducted by Japanese Society of Anesthesiologists. *Masui* 2003; **52**: 304–19.

Section 3

Subspeciality in Anesthesiology

Chapter 3

Anesthesia for Urological Surgery

Zeki Tuncel Tekgül, Burcu Özalp Horsanali and Mustafa Ozan Horsanali

Additional information is available at the end of the chapter

http://dx.doi.org/10.5772/66196

Abstract

Because of the variable techniques and patients' positions used in urological surgery, anesthesia for urologic surgery requires advanced knowledge and special transactions. In this matter, it is important to follow current approaches for anesthesiologists. Different surgical procedures and complications due to different positions or anesthesia were evaluated separately to be more concise. We have researched recent literature and created this chapter about new technologies in urological surgery and development in anesthesia for urological surgery.

Keywords: urological anesthesia, anesthesia management, anesthesia complications, urological surgery complications

1. Introduction

Anesthesia for urological surgery includes unique distinctive differences, as in all other surgical departments. Therefore, anesthesia for urological surgery requires featured training and experience.

To reduce the risk of complications in urological surgery, like all other kinds of surgery, regional anesthesia techniques came to prominence with the help of technological developments. For many urological ventures, only neuraxial blockade application could be enough. This also results in decreased complication risks. In surgeries that must be done with general anesthesia, epidural anesthesia can be used for the maintenance of anesthesia or in the postoperative period. In this way, the rate of intraoperative complications can be reduced and patients' comfort can be increased by providing postoperative pain control and also duration of hospital stay can be reduced [1].

During the urological surgery, different complications can develop depending on surgical techniques used. For example, most of urological ventures require lots of irrigation fluids. In this venture, use of unheated irrigation fluid can lead to complications such as hypothermia, delayed recovery from anesthesia and tremor [2].

In addition to neuraxial blockade, the use of peripheral blockade has gained importance in urological surgery. For example, obturator blockade application for lateral wall localized bladder cancer could reduce intraoperative complications and increased cancer-free survival [3, 4].

2. Anesthesia for kidney and upper urinary tract surgery

2.1. Oncological surgery of kidney and upper urinary tract

2.1.1. Radical and partial nephrectomy

Renal cell carcinoma (RCC) is the ninth common cancer in the USA. According to the SEER database analysis, it is estimated that there will be 62,700 new cases and 14,240 people will die because of this disease. The incidence of kidney and renal pelvis cancer was 15.6 per 100,000 in the USA between 2009 and 2013 [5]. All around the world, radical or partial nephrectomy is accepted curative treatment for kidney tumors. Partial nephrectomy can be performed depending on the tumor size and localization of tumor. During the partial nephrectomy, localized solid mass must be removed entirely with clear surgical margins [6]. The European Association of Urology (EAU) Renal Cell Cancer Guidelines Panel recommends partial nephrectomy for the tumors less than 4 cm [7].

The flank incision provides advantages in terms of access to the kidney directly, but in case of vena cava involvement, it can be insufficient anatomically. If the tumor size is huge and abdomen exploration or contralateral retroperitoneal exploration is needed, subcostal incision may supply advantages to the surgeon. Various factors including surgeon's experience, tumor size and localization, patient's body habits and localization of affected kidney can affect the incision type [8].

2.1.2. Radical nephroureterectomy

Upper urothelial cell carcinoma is a rare tumor among genitourinary system tumors that constitute approximately 5% [9]. Radical nephroureterectomy with bladder cuff resections is a standard curative treatment for patients with non-metastatic upper urothelial cell carcinoma, although advanced developments of minimal invasive surgery and surgical techniques for radical surgery are present [10].

2.1.2.1. Preoperative considerations

Known risk factors for RCC include tobacco smoking and be over the age of 60. The peak incidence of RCC is at the age of 60 years and male-female ratio is 2:1. Hence, these patients with RCC generally have comorbidities such as coronary-after-disease and chronic obstructive pulmonary disease. Only small percent of patients (approximately 10%) have classic diagnostic triad of symptoms including flank pain, hematuria and palpable abdominal mass. Paraneoplastic symptoms and impaired laboratory test including increased erythrocyte sedimentation rate, eosinophilia and increased hormone levels of prolactin, renin and glucocorticoids [11]. The patient's health status is also optimized by management of anemia, glycemic control and treatment for hypertension, as well as dietary, weight and smoking-cessation advice before surgery. A consultant-led, multidisciplinary decision can be made as to which procedure and approach are required for each patient [12]. Because these patients usually have comorbid disease such as advanced age, hypertension, diabetes, chronic obstructive pulmonary disease and congestive heart failure and they have had a long and major surgery, it should be appropriate to prepare intensive care bed for these patients to stay in intensive care unit for the critical postoperative period. Intensive care unit can be appropriate to follow up and interfere with postoperative problems that must be treated quickly such as hypothermia, electrolyte imbalance, hemorrhage, infections, pulmonary disorders and requirement of dialysis.

2.1.2.2. Intraoperative considerations

In thoraco-abdominal approach, since the pleural space is entered, using the noble-lumen endotracheal tube may facilitate the surgery by deflating the ipsilateral lung. Postoperative ventilation may be needed because of prolonged retraction of the lung that is causing contusion. During the diaphragm dissection, the phrenic nerve may also be injured by both thoraco-abdominal incision and flank incision. During operation, excessive blood loss may occur at any stage of operation, which is the reason for the high vascularity of the tumor. Bleeding can be caused by the surrenal gland. At last, adjacent abdominal organs including colon, duodenum and liver may be injured. If the renal mass is on the left side, bleeding due to splenic injury may occur with an incidence as high as 10% [13]. When extensive bleeding is observed, wide-channel venous cannulation and central venous cannulation should be obtained for monitoring both the central venous pressure and supply rapid blood transfusion. Prolonged retraction of vena cava may result of transient hypotension. Hence, direct arterial pressure monitoring may facilitate the control of blood pressure, especially in patients with cardiac comorbidity. Moreover, these applications may be helpful for the patients who need mechanic ventilation postoperatively. If the patient has caval obstruction due to naval thrombus, additional management may be needed. Embolization of the tumor fragment may occur during the central venous catheter application, if the thrombus in vena cava extends into the right atrium. When atrial thrombus is observed, a pulmonary artery catheter is contraindicated. For this reason, many authors suggested that the use of intraoperative transesophageal echocardiography in order to detect tumor extension in the inferior vena cava [14–16].

2.1.2.3. Choice of anesthesia

The anesthetic management of patients undergoing radical nephrectomy should include general endotracheal anesthesia. Alternately, combined regional/general endotracheal anesthesia advised to be employed. If the general and epidural anesthesia are combined, epidural catheter must be placed and test dose should be administered before the induction of general anesthesia. To perform the induction of general anesthesia after evaluating the effect of the test dose will be reduced the risk of unintended intrathecal and intravascular injection. Although test dose is administered, it would be safer to administer the epidural dose partially and intermittently. When neuraxial blockade performed, sensorial block level must be Th4. It has been shown that intraoperative epidural infusion of local anesthetic suppresses the stress hormone response and reduces opioid requirement when compared to straight general anesthesia in open nephrectomy [13]. Also, it is advised to reduce pulmonary complications and be more effective to control postoperative pain.

2.1.2.4. Complications

Patients with renal failure may be sensitive to benzodiazepines. Cisatracurium may be considered for muscle relaxation as it is metabolized via ester hydrolysis and Hofmann elimination. Other pharmacologic considerations for the patient with renal failure include adjusted dosing of antibiotics and avoidance of nonsteroidal anti-inflammatory agents. Patients with chronic kidney failure have decreased platelet function and von Willebrand factor and reduced red blood cell volume. So the anesthesiologist must transfuse appropriate blood product [17].

2.2. Nononcological surgery of kidney and upper urinary tract

Nononcological urological surgery of kidney and upper urinary tract includes such procedures like simple nephrectomy, pyeloplasty, nephrolithotomy or pyelolithotomy, percutaneous nephrolithotomy (PNL), extracorporeal shockwave lithotripsy (ESWL), retrograde intrarenal surgery (RIRS), percutaneous nephrostomy, ureterorenoscopy and ureteral stent replacement. Open stone surgery (nephrolithotomy or pyelolithotomy) is now dramatically reducing and the endoscopic and extracorporeal methods are increasing, overcoat ESWL in those hospitals which has an own lithotripter. Open surgery is actually indicated for the complex renal stone and the complicated ureteral stone [18]. Classically, PNL is done on the patient first in the supine position for replacement of the ureteral catheter and then in a prone position for accessing the caliceal system. Other procedures such as simple nephrectomy, pyeloplasty, nephrolithotomy and pyelolithotomy are performed on the patients in the lateral decubitus position.

2.2.1. Preoperative considerations

The anesthesiologist should evaluate not only patients' history and physical examination but also existing urinary tract infection. If it exists, antibiotherapy must be given perioperatively. All anticoagulation medications including aspirin and nonsteroidal anti-inflammatory drugs (NSAIDs) are typically held for 5 days prior to surgery. Blood type and screening are recommended for the patients who are at high risk of intraoperative bleeding.

2.2.2. Intraoperative considerations

Antegrade or retrograde ureteropyelography (RPG) is often used to demonstrate the anatomical structure of urinary system or localized the level of urinary system obstruction. Due to the radiographic-iodinated contrast media used in such PNL procedure, patients have predisposed factors for iodinated contrast media-related adverse reactions such as a previous adverse reaction to iodinated contrast media, a history of asthma and atopy, dehydration, acute or chronic renal diseases and advanced age, where iodinated contrast media-induced adverse reactions may observed [19]. The prone position alone for PNL is associated with a variety of position-related complications. To avoid cervical spine injury during positioning, the head should be held in a neutral position through the turn and positioning. Neck extension or head rotation could also impede carotid and/or vertebral artery blood flow and venous return. The etiology of peripheral nerve injury is usually multifactorial, requiring both a direct pressure and a stretch component. The large volume of irrigation fluid used during PCNL can decrease body temperature. Hence, monitoring core temperature is routine [2, 20, 21].

2.2.3. Choice of anesthesia

Commonly, general anesthesia with an endotracheal intubation is preferred for simple nephrectomy, pyeloplasty, nephrolithotomy, pyelolithotomy and PNL, although sedation and neuraxial anesthesia for PNL have also been successful [22]. If neuraxial blockade is performed, the sensorial block level must be Th4.

Recently, anesthetic management of routine ESWL treatments on adults covers effective sedative and analgesic practice. Different applications could be used successfully such as meperidine and promethazine, midazolam with alfentanil, fentanyl and ketamine. Substantial research on the use of alfentanil by various routes reported that this drug is very effective [23–25].

2.2.4. Complications

The major complications during nononcological urological surgery of kidney and upper urinary system tract includes bleeding, bowel and collecting system injury, traumatic arteriovenous fistula or false aneurysm, sepsis, atelectasis, pneumothorax, pleural effusion and hemothorax [26, 27]. As excessive amount of irrigation solution is used intraoperatively in surgical procedures like PCNL, hypothermia is frequently observed. Tekgül and colleagues reported that effects of irrigation solutions, administered at either 21 or 37°C in percutaneous nephrolithotomy (PCNL), on hypothermia and related postoperative complications such as late emergence and late recovery from anesthesia, shivering, lactic acidosis and excess bleeding [2].

3. Anesthesia for bladder and prostate

3.1. Oncological surgery of bladder and prostate

This part covers transurethral resection of bladder tumor (TUR BT), radical cystectomy and radical prostatectomy operations as urological surgery. Bladder cancer is the fourth most common cancer in the United States. Initial diagnosis and treatment of non-muscle invasive bladder cancer is TUR BT. Radical cystectomy is the treatment of choice for invasive urinary bladders tumors. Prostate cancer is a major cause of morbidity and mortality and it is estimated that there will be 240,890 new diagnoses of prostate cancer in 2011 and that prostate cancer will be responsible for approximately 33,720 deaths in 2011 [28].

3.1.1. Preoperative considerations

Average blood loss associated with radical cystectomy has been reported from 560 to 3000 mL [29, 30] and blood loss associated with radical retropubic prostatectomy is commonly reported between 550 and 800 mL, although higher estimates are infrequently reported [31, 32]. Blood transfusion for patients with high risk of bleeding has been recommended before elective procedures.

In patients who underwent surgery, the major and most common causes of the nonsurgical death are deep vein thrombosis (DVT) and related pulmonary thromboembolism. Especially, patients who underwent radical surgery such as prostatectomy and cystectomy have major risk factors for development of DVT due to malignancy, surgery, immobility and advanced age. For good postoperative care of patients and to prevent the development of DVT, DVT profilaxy is needed before the surgery in patients with high risk for DVT. The risk of development DVT in patients undergoing open radical prostatectomy without DVT profilaxy is estimated to be 32% [33].

3.1.2. Intraoperative considerations

Because of the possible excessive blood loss, wide-channel venous cannula is required. After positioning the patient, arterial cannula should be placed for monitoring the patient. If there is a risk for excessive blood loss, central venous catheter should be utilized for purpose of transfusion. However, central venous pressure monitoring could not demonstrate cardiac performance related to fluid infusion [34].

3.1.3. Choice of anesthesia

General endotracheal anesthesia is indicated; consideration should be given to a combined general/neuraxial technique for postoperative analgesia [35]. The sensorial block level must be Th10 for TUR BT and Th6 for radical cystectomy or prostatectomy. Especially, obturator nerve blockade should be added to neuraxial block to prevent the adductor jerk due to electrical stimulation of cautery applied in lateral wall localized tumors of the bladder. Obturator nerve block is performed following verification of the level of spinal anesthesia with the patient in lithotomy position. A 21 gauge 100 mm stimulable needle is inserted perpendicularly 2 cm inferior and 2 cm lateral point from the pubic tubercle. According to the "traditional approach", the needle was inserted from the skin through the inferior rami of the pubic bone, redirected anterolaterally and contacting with the obturator nerve after advancing to a depth of 2–4 cm. After the contraction of adductor muscle group was observed, 10 mL 0.25% levobupivacaine was administered with current at 0.3–0.5 mA [3, 4].

3.1.4. Complications

The anesthesiologist should always consider that patients underwent radical cystectomy and urinary diversion could produce bacteremia. If ileal conduit operation performed, ionic alterations may cause metabolic disturbances. This disorder usually emerges in the form of hyperchloremic metabolic acidosis. When urine contact with intestinal segment, ammonium, ammonia, hydrogen and chloride are reabsorbed from intestinal segment. Alkalizing agents or drugs such as chlorpromazine or nicotinic acid that blockade the chloride transport can be used successfully for the treatment of this disorder [35].

Hemorrhage is the most common observed complication of radical surgery in urological field. For radical prostatectomy operations during the pelvic lymph node dissection hypogastric veins can be injured and results in extensive blood loss. Similarly, the deep dorsal vein complex can be injured during the transection of this vein complex and extensive blood loss may also occur. Additionally, deep vein thrombosis and pulmonary thromboembolism are other radical prostatectomy-related major complications [30].

3.2. Nononcological surgery of bladder and prostate

Nononcological urological surgery procedures of bladder and prostate include such as transurethral resection of prostate, suprapubic transvesical prostatectomy and cystoscopy. Most patients with bladder obstruction caused by benign prostatic hyperplasia are successfully treated by transurethral resection of the prostate (TURP) or, if prostate size is over than 70 cc, suprapubic transvesical prostatectomy could be performed [36]. Diagnostic examination of the lower urinary tract is often performed using a cystoscope and initial diagnosis and treatment of bladder cancer is conducted by transurethral resection of bladder.

3.2.1. Preoperative considerations

This procedure is often performed on older patients with impaired renal function, cardiovascular and respiratory problems. Thus, it is important to limit the block level to minimize hemodynamic changes during the spinal anesthesia in such patients [37, 38].

3.2.2. Intraoperative considerations

During the resection of prostate, surgeon must take maximum care not to damage prostatic capsule. In 2% of the patients who underwent resection of the prostate, capsule perforation may occur. In these patients, symptoms such as restlessness, nausea, vomiting and abdominal pain can be observed. If perforation occurred, the operation must be terminated immediately [39]. Bleeding may occur during the TURP but can be controlled easily. Since the irrigation fluids and blood mix during the TURP, it is difficult to determine the amount of bleeding. According to the researches, estimated bleeding during the TURP operation is 2–4 mL/min of resection time or 20–50 mL/g of resected prostatic tissue [40]. The need for transfusion due to hemorrhage during TURP is in 2.5% of patients undergoing TURP [41].

The clinical presentation of TURP syndrome is multifactorial, initiated by excessive absorption of irrigating solution that affects central nerve system (CNS), cardiovascular, respiratory and metabolic homeostasis. Initial signs of TURP syndrome cover burning sensations in the face and neck along with lethargy and apprehension. Additionally, headache and irritability may be observed due to affected CNS. Finally, visual disturbances, confusion, seizures and eventually coma may be observed. These CNS disturbances have been attributed to hyponatremia, which occurs with the absorption of any type of irrigating solution and hyperglycinemia and/or hyperammonemia if glycine is used [42, 43]. The amount and rate of fluid absorption depend on several factors such as hydrostatic pressure of the irrigation fluids, bladder distention, the size of opened venous sinuses and the length of resection time [44]. If there is a suspicion of TURP syndrome, operation must be terminated immediately and blood samples including electrolytes, creatinine, glucose and arterial blood gases must be sent for analyses and electrocardiogram should be obtained [45]. Treatment of hyponatremia and excessive fluid loading should be adjusted according to the severity of the patient's symptoms. When patient's symptoms are mild (serum sodium level is greater than 120 mEq/L), only fluid restriction combined with loop diuretics can be enough to bring increased serum sodium levels to normal levels. If the serum sodium levels are less than 120 mEq/L, intravenous hypertonic saline administration is recommended for the patients with severe symptoms. The 3% sodium chloride solution 100 mL/h should be infused and the patient's serum sodium levels should be corrected at a rate not greater than 0.5 mEq/L/h [46, 47].

3.2.3. *Choice of anesthesia*

Sedation and routine patient monitoring is enough for minor procedures. But other procedures such as suprapubic transvesical prostatectomy and TURP or necessitate full distension of the bladder, a neuraxial anesthesia should be used. The block level must be Th10.

3.2.4. *Complications*

Bleeding, transurethral resection syndrome (TUR), bladder perforation, hypothermia, intraoperative and early postoperative occurrence of disseminated intravascular coagulation are most common observed complications of TURP. Providing stable anesthesia is essential for these patients to minimize hemodynamic changes. Under the general anesthesia, it could be difficult to realize complications such as TUR syndrome and bladder perforation, so regional anesthesia is recommended for TURP operations [48, 49]. Side effects of TUR BT is bladder perforation that has a reported incidence of 0.9–5% and presents with the signs and symptoms of inability to distend the bladder, low return of irrigation solution, abdominal distension and tachycardia [50]. Rarely, intraperitoneal fluid extravasation related to bladder perforation during the TUR BT can be identified as 'TUR BT syndrome'. Similar clinic symptoms can be observed like TUR P syndrome, but in TUR BT syndrome, intravascular fluid deficit that causes renal impairment is not observed. The mechanism of the possible causes of intravascular hypovolemia is that sodium equilibrates with the intraperitoneal fluid [51]. If the tumoral mass localized near the obturator nerve in bladder wall, bladder perforation may occur during the resection. The obturator nerve usually passes through the pelvis close to the lateral bladder wall, bladder neck and prostatic urethra. During the resection of bladder cancer, obturator nerve may stimulated by electrocautery that causes bladder perforation by the forceful thigh contraction of adductor muscles. Recently, combined neuraxial and obturator nerve blockage is recommended to prevent this complication. This combined technique is recommended to reduce the complications of general anesthesia in these patients which often covers older patients with lots of comorbidities.

http://dx.doi.org/10.5772/66196

4. Anesthesia for urethra and genital surgery

4.1. Oncological surgery of genital legion

In this section, the title of oncologic surgery of the genital region covers the operations of radical orchiectomy and retroperitoneal lymph node dissection. Initial treatment of testicular cancer is radical orchiectomy with inguinal incision. Retroperitoneal lymph node dissection (RPLND) for the treatment of testicular cancer is a relatively rare and complex operation after chemotherapy.

4.1.1. Preoperative consideration

The preoperative medical evaluation of cancer patients should include an assessment of nutritional status, functional status and symptom control (particularly regarding cancer-related pain) in addition to an assessment of general medical issues. The natural history of the cancer and effects of any prior chemotherapy or radiation therapy should also be considered [52].

Pulmonary insufficiency may occur in patients who underwent retroperitoneal lymph node dissection and have adjuvant bleomycin preoperatively. Oxygen toxicity and fluid overload may also develop, too. Physicians must be careful in terms of developing acute respiratory distress syndrome postoperatively for these patients.

4.1.2. Intraoperative consideration

Routine monitorization of the patient is enough. If bradycardia occurs, surgeon must be warned to reduce the stretch of the spermatic cord and if it does not improve, 1 mg atropin should be given.

4.1.3. Choice of anesthesia

Neuraxial anesthesia has been considered as the anesthetic technique of choice for radical orchiectomy. Sensorial block level must be Th10, but minimized to psychiatric trauma, sedation must be added to neuraxial blockade. For the RPLND procedure general anesthesia must be chosen. If neuraxial blockade is chosen (if general anesthesia is contraindicated), high-level sensorial block (Th4) with sedation must be performed.

4.1.4. Complications

Sometimes in this procedure, vagal reflex and bradycardia can occur during the operation due to stretch of the spermatic cord and patient can feel pain.

4.2. Nononcological surgery of urethra and genital legion

This section covers urological procedures such as cystoscopy, urethrotomy interna, scrotal orchiectomy, hydrocelectomy, varicocelectomy and penile prosthesis implantation.

4.2.1. Preoperative consideration

These procedures generally do not require any particular anesthetic technique, depending upon the procedure, the medical condition of the patient and patient's and/or surgeon's preference, one technique may be more appropriate.

4.2.2. Intraoperative consideration

Routine monitorization is advised. During the varicocelectomy, bradycardia can occur due to stretch of the spermatic cord.

4.2.3. Choice of anesthesia

Many of these procedures are ambulatory, performed in cystoscopy suites with a rapid turnover of patients and the anesthetic choice must also consider these concerns. Evaluation of the lower urinary system tract is often performed by the urologist with a flexible cystoscope. This procedure generally performed by the urologist with local topical anesthesia applied to the inside of the urethra as it does not require full bladder distention. If patient could not tolerate pain, the procedure must be performed under monitored anesthesia care with sedation [53]. Neuraxial anesthesia has been long considered the anesthetic technique of choice for these urological procedures. The sensorial block level must be Th10.

4.2.4. Complications

During the varicocelectomy, bradycardia can occur due to stretch of the spermatic cord.

5. Anesthesia for urological laparoscopic surgery

Laparoscopic procedures in urology cover both oncological surgery like nephrectomy, prostatectomy, cystectomy and nononcological surgery like pyeloplasty. Laparoscopic surgery has found wide applications in urological surgery with the developing technology. After laparoscopic surgery, some complications due to pneumoperitoneum began to occur more frequent.

5.1. Preoperative considerations

An anesthetic plan is developed based not only on the patient's physical status determined by the assessment but on how the patient will tolerate pneumoperitoneum and body position during the surgery. Some factors like obesity and Trendelenburg level may increase the intraabdominal pressure during the laparoscopic operations. These factors should be considered, when anesthetic management is planned. Difficult airway, cardiopulmonary status, allergies, medications and comorbid conditions are important issues for patients undergoing laparoscopic surgery. Especially, decision of laparoscopic surgery should be considered carefully in patients with advanced respiratory disorder because of the high risk of anesthesia.

5.2. Intraoperative considerations

Pneumoperitoneum and patient positioning impede normal respiratory mechanics. Placement of an endotracheal tube allows the ventilator to supply the work necessary to breathe. Gastric secretions are commonly seen in the oropharynx or on the face of patients at the end of surgery. The placement of an arterial line may be indicated if the patient's medical condition warrants closer blood pressure monitoring nasogastric tube decompression of the stomach and Foley catheter drainage of the bladder is the basic procedure for most urologic laparoscopic surgeries. Hypothermia is common beginning with the disruption of thermal regulation due to anesthesia.

5.3. Choice of anesthesia

Most common anesthetic plan is general anesthesia. General endotracheal anesthesia is chosen to counter the adverse conditions created by the pneumoperitoneum, patient positioning and surgical time. If general anesthesia is contraindicated, high level sensorial block (Th4) can be performed.

5.4. Complications

Anesthetic complications are addressed through that prism: anesthetic strategies to minimize hemodynamic changes due to pneumoperitoneum and patient position. Increasing the intrathoracic blood volume improved hemodynamic function in all body positions with pneumoperitoneum. Fluid management is the most important element for minimizing pneumoperitoneum side effects [54].

Most common observed complications of laparoscopic surgeries are swelling of the face, eyelids, conjunctivae and tongue along with a plethoric color of venous stasis in the head and neck. Although facial edema is common, but laryngeal edema may prevent the extubation of patient and can cause delay extubation in 5% of patients [55, 56].

6. Anesthesia for urologic emergency

Urologic emergencies requiring surgical intervention are relatively rare. This section reviews both the common and rare urologic emergencies such as renal trauma, bladder trauma, urethral trauma, scrotal trauma, testicular torsion and fournier gangrene.

Testicular torsion occurs due to rotation of spermatic cord around. This rotation blocks the blood flow of testis and impairs venous drainage. As a result of this pathology, edema, ischemia and necrosis develop. Testicular torsion is common in the two periods of life. While first peak is at age of 1–2 years, second peak is common in adolescence. Testicular torsion is rarely observed after the age of 40 [57].

6.1. Preoperative considerations

In patients with fournier gangrene, there is usually rapid development of severe toxemia leading to sepsis and progressive organ dysfunction. The appropriate administration of intravenous fluid therapy to maintain an effective circulating volume and prevent and inadequate tissue perfusion is a core element of the preoperative practice of the anesthesia [58].

6.2. Intraoperative considerations

Routine monitorization is advised for all patients with urological emergencies. The patient with the risk of hypovolemia and hypotension, central venous catheterization must be performed to monitor the central venous pressure and providing rapid fluid transfusion. Invasive arterial blood pressure must be done to follow blood pressure in patients with the risk of hypotension.

6.3. Choice of anesthesia

Most common anesthetic plan is general anesthesia in trauma patients, but neuraxial blockade can be chosen for testicular torsion. If effected area is localized in patients with fournier gangrene or the patient is not septic, neuraxial blockade can be chosen, too. The sensorial block level must be chosen according to the level of legion. Th10 sensorial block level can be enough for testicular torsion.

7. Patient positioning for urological surgery

Nerve injuries comprise 22% of all anesthesia-related medico-legal claims in the United States [59]. In an extensive study that reviewed 380,680 cases over 10 years in single center reported that perioperative nerve injuries were observed in 112 cases. Urological procedures were 15% of all cases and 13% of cases have peripheral nerve injuries [60].

Different ocular injuries can be observed. Although minor complications like corneal abrasion that can occur in any position are common, major complications like ischemic optic neuropathy occur in prone or Trendelenburg positions [61]. Compartment syndrome has been reported to occur in several positions after prolonged urologic surgery [62].

7.1. The supine position

The upper extremities should be properly secured to avoid pressure on the ulnar groove or hyperextension. One or both arms may be adducted or abducted while supine. Padding should be placed over the elbow and any sharp objects and the arms secured using the draw sheet tucked underneath the patient rather than the mattress.

Ulnar neuropathy is the most frequent site (28%) of anesthesia-related nerve injury according to the ASA Closed Claims Database [63]. The median nerve is susceptible to neuropathy due to excessive stretching as it courses through the antecubital fossa. Careful attention should be given to avoid hyperextension at the elbow [64].

7.2. The prone position

It is most commonly used for percutaneous nephrolithotomy, adrenalectomy and pediatric pyeloplasty via the dorsal lumbotomy approach. During positioning, attention should be paid to avoid inadvertent extubation of the trachea and to maintain the neck in neutral position, fixed relative to the thorax. All pressure points, including forehead, chin, elbows, knees, shins and toes, must be properly padded.

A decrease in cardiac index (CI) can occur when turning patients from the supine to the prone position ranging from 12.9 to 24% [20].

In contrast to the supine position, the prone position results in a minimal reduction in functional residual capacity relative to the upright position [65].

Other rare complications related to the prone position are ophthalmic injury, upper airway edema and venous air embolism.

7.3. The lithotomy position

The lithotomy position is most frequently used for transurethral cystoscopy procedures or for open urologic procedures where access to the perineum and anus is necessary. Elevating the legs into the lithotomy position translocates the blood volume of the lower extremities into the central compartment, increasing venous return. Similar to the supine position, placing the legs into lithotomy position will shift the abdominal viscera cephalad into the diaphragm, decreasing lung capacities and compliance.

Neuropathy of the common peroneal nerve is the most common lower extremity neuropathy seen in the lithotomy position, accounting for 78% of lower extremity nerve injuries [66]. The obturator nerve, which supplies motor innervation to thigh adductors, may be stretched when the patient's hips are flexed beyond 80–100° [67]. Posterior tibial nerve, lateral femoral cutaneous nerve and saphaneus nerve can be injured during lithotomy position.

7.4. The Trendelenburg position

The Trendelenburg position is obtained by tilting the patient in the supine position to head down. According to the Trendelenburg position, abdominal organs move toward the diaphragm and facilitate the exploration of lower abdomen and pelvis by surgeons. The arms should be abducted <90° in the neutral position preferably. Physicians should be careful about the sliding down of the arms from the board when patient is tilted [68].

The Trendelenburg position may cause visual loss by impairing the venous drainage of the head. If the patient's head below the level of the heart, increased intracranial and venous pressure can intensify the pressure on optic nerve [69].

Edema can be observed in head or neck, due to the increased intracranial and venous pressure caused by the prolonged Trendelenburg position. Swelling of the face, eyes, larynx and tongue may occur and is essential for indication of fluid resuscitation.

7.5. The lateral decubitus position

The lateral decubitus position generally is preferred to explore surreal gland, kidney or collecting system without entering the peritoneal space. This position is suitable for simple nephrectomy procedure, removing renal tones that required open surgery and ureter stones localized in the upper urinary system.

Cardiac output while in the lateral decubitus position should remain unchanged unless venous return is impeded. Ventilation is increased in the dependent lung and gas exchange remains unchanged [70].

Author details

Zeki Tuncel Tekgül[1]*, Burcu Özalp Horsanali[1] and Mustafa Ozan Horsanali[2]

*Address all correspondence to: zekittekgul@yahoo.com

1 Department of Anesthesiology and Reanimation, Izmir Bozyaka Research and Training Hospital, Izmir, Turkey

2 Department of Urology, Izmir Atatürk Research and Training Hospital, Izmir, Turkey

References

[1] Hammady A, Abdelgalil W, Rashed E, Elbadry MS. Upper urinary tract retroperitoneoscopic surgery under epidural anesthesia: Shifting towards outpatient treatment. Scand J Urol. 2015;49(2):181–184.

[2] Tekgül ZT, Pektas S, Yildirim U, Karaman Y, Cakmak M, Ozkarakas H, Gonullu M. A prospective randomized double-blind study on the effects of the temperature of irrigation solutions on thermoregulation and postoperative complications in percutaneous nephrolithotomy. J Anesth. 2015;29:165–169.

[3] Tekgül ZT, Divrik RT, Turan M, Konyalioğlu E, Simsek E, Gönüllü M. Impact of obturator nerve block on the short-term recurrence of superficial bladder tumors on the lateral wall. Urol J. 2014;11(1):1249–1252.

[4] Bolat D, Aydogdu O, Tekgul ZT, Polat S, Yonguc T, Bozkurt IH, Sen V, Okur O. Impact of nerve stimulator-guided obturator nerve block on the short-term outcomes and complications of transurethral resection of bladder tumour: A prospective randomized controlled study. Can Urol Assoc J. 2015;9(11–12):780–784.

[5] Howlader N, Noone AM, Krapcho M, Miller D, Bishop K, Altekruse SF, Kosary CL, Yu M, Ruhl J, Tatalovich Z, Mariotto A, Lewis DR, Chen HS, Feuer EJ, Cronin KA (eds). SEER Cancer Statistics Review, 1975–2013. Bethesda, MD: National Cancer Institute; 2016. http://seer.cancer.gov/csr/1975_2013/, based on November 2015 SEER data submission, posted to the SEER web site.

[6] Uzzo R, Novick A. Nephron sparing surgery for renal tumors: Indications, techniques and outcomes. J Urol. 2001;166:6–18.

[7] Ljungberg B, Bensalah K, Bex A, Canfield S, Dabestani S, Hofmann F, et al. EAU guidelines on renal cell carcinoma. 2015;67(5):913–24.

[8] Whalley DG, Berrigan MJ. Anesthesia for radical prostatectomy, cystectomy, nephrectomy, pheochromocytoma and laparoscopic procedures. Anesthesiol Clin North Am. 2000;18(4):899–991.

[9] Jemal A, Siegel R, Ward E, Hao Y, Xu J, Thun MJ. Cancer statistics, 2009. CA Cancer J Clin. 2009;59:225–249.

[10] Babjuk M, Burger M, Zigeuner R, et al. EAU guidelines on non-muscle-invasive urothelial carcinoma of the bladder: Update 2013. Eur Urol. 2013;64:639–653.

[11] Garnick MB. Bladder, renal and testicular cancer. In: Dale DC, Federman DD, editors. Scientific American Medicine. New York: Scientific American; 1999.

[12] Cockcroft JOB, Berry CB, McGrath JS, Mark O. Anesthesia for major urologic surgery. Anesthesiol Clin. 2015;33:165–172.

[13] Li Y. Combined general/epidural anesthesia (ropivacaine 0.375%) versus general anesthesia for upper abdominal surgery. Anesth Analg. 2008;106(5):1562–1565.

[14] Hasnain JU, Watson RJN. Transesophageal echocardiography during resection of renal cell carcinoma involving the inferior vena cava. South Med J. 1994;87:273–275.

[15] Mizoguchi T, Koide Y, Ohara M, et al. Multiplane transesophageal echocardiographic guidance during resection of renal cell carcinoma extending in the inferior vena cava. Anesth Analg. 1995;81:1102–1105.

[16] Ohara J, Sprung J, Whalley D, et al. Transesophageal echocardiography in monitoring of intrapulmonary embolism during inferior vena cava tumor resection. J Cardiothorac Vasc Anesth. 1999;13:69–71.

[17] Dorgalaleh A, Mahmudi M, Tabibian S, Khatib ZK, Tamaddon GH, Moghaddam ES, Bamedi T, Alizadeh S, Moradi E. Anemia and thrombocytopenia in acute and chronic renal failure. Int J Hematol Oncol Stem Cell Res. 2013;7(4):34–39.

[18] González Enguita C, Calahorra Fernández FJ, Cabrera Pérez J, García Cardoso J, Rodríguez-Miñón Cifuentes JL, García de la Peña E, et al. Surgery of renoureteral lithiasis. Current indications. Actas Urol Esp. 2001;25(9):610–617.

[19] Meth MJ, Maibach HI. Current understanding of contrast media reactions and implications for clinical management. Drug Saf. 2006;29:133–141.

[20] Edgcombe H, Carter K, Yarrow S. Anaesthesia in the prone position. Br J Anaesth. 2008;100:165–183.

[21] Rozentsveig V, Neulander AZ, Roussabrov E, et al. Anesthetic considerations during percutaneous nephrolithotomy. J Clin Anesth. 2007;19:351–355.

[22] Aravantinos E, Karatzas A, Gravas S, Tzortizs V. Feasibility of percutaneous nephrolithotomy under assisted local anaesthesia: A prospective study on selected patients with upper urinary tract obstruction. Eur Urol. 2007;51:224–228.

[23] Morgulis R, Yarmush J, Woglom J, et al. Alfentanil analgesia/sedation for extracorporeal shock wave lithotripsy: A comparison with general and epidural anesthesia. AANA J. 1991;59:533–537.

[24] McCullough DL. Extracorporeal shock wave lithotripsy. In: Walsh PC, Retic AB, Stamey TA, et al., editors. Campbell's Urology. Philadelphia: WB Saunders; 1992. pp. 2168–2177.

[25] Chin CM, Tay KP, Lim PHC, et al. Use of patient-controlled analgesia in extracorporeal shockwave lithotripsy. Br J Urol. 1997;79:848–851.

[26] Giusti G, Piccinelli A, Taverna G, et al. Miniperc? No, thank you! Eur Urol. 2007;51:810–815.

[27] Zagoria RJ, Dyer RB. Do's and don'ts of percutaneous nephrostomy. Acad Radiol. 1999;6:370–377.

[28] Howlader N, Noone A, Krapcho M, et al. SEER Cancer Statistics Review, 1975–2008. Bethesda: National Cancer Institute; 2010. SEER data submission, posted on the SEER web site, 2011.

[29] Soulie M, Straub M, Game X, et al. A multicenter study of the morbidity of radical cystectomy in select elderly patients with bladder cancer. J Urol. 2002;167:1325–1328.

[30] Knap N, Lundbeck F, Overguard J. Early and late treatment-related morbidity following radical cystectomy. Scand J Urol Nephrol. 2005;39:153–160.

[31] Jurczok A, Zacharias M, Wagner S, et al. Prospective non-randomized evaluation of four mediators of the systemic response after extraperitoneal laparoscopic and open retropubic radical prostatectomy. BJU Int. 2007;99(6):1461–1466.

[32] Rocco B, Matei DV, Melegari S, et al. Robotic vs open prostatectomy in a laparoscopically naïve centre: a matched-pair analysis. BJU Int. 2009;104(7):991–995.

[33] Nicolaides AN, Breddin HK, Fareed J, Goldhaber S, Haas S, Hull R, et al. Cardiovascular Disease Educational and Research Trust and the International Union of Angiology. Prevention of venous thromboembolism. International Consensus Statement. Guidelines compiled in accordance with the scientific evidence. 2001;20(1):1–37.

[34] Kumar A, Anel R, Bunnell E, et al. Pulmonary artery occlusion pressure and central venous pressure fail to predict ventricular filling volume, cardiac performance, or the response to volume infusion in normal subjects. Crit Care Med. 2004;32:691–699.

[35] Maffezzini M, Campodonico F, Canepa G, et al. Current perioperative management of radical cystectomy with intestinal urinary reconstruction for muscle-invasive bladder cancer and reduction of the incidence of postoperative ileus. Surg Oncol. 2008;17:41–48.

[36] Van der Aa F, Joniau S, Van Den Dranden M, et al. Metabolic changes after urinary diversion. Adv Urol. 2011;2001:Article ID 764325, p. 5.

[37] Mebust WK, Holtgrewe HL, Cockett ATK, Peters PC. Transurethral prostatectomy: Immediate and postoperative complications-a cooperative study of 13 participating institutions evaluating 3,885 patients. J Urol. 2002;167:5–9.

[38] Kim SY, Cho JE, Hong JY, Koo BN, Kim JM, Kil HK. Comparison of intrathecal fentanyl and sufentanil in low-dose dilute bupivacaine spinal anaesthesia for transurethral prostatectomy. Br J Anaesth. 2009;103:750–754.

[39] Azar I. Transurethral prostatectomy syndrome and other complications of urological procedures. In: McLeskey CH, editor. Geriatric Anesthesia. 1st ed. Baltimore: Williams & Wilkins; 1997. pp. 595–607.

[40] Fitzpatrick JM, Mebust WK. Minimally invasive and endoscopic management of benign prostatic hyperplasia. In: Walsh PC, editor. Campbell's Urology. 8th ed. Philadelphia: WB Saunders; 2002. pp. 1379–1422.

[41] Hatch PD. Surgical and anaesthetic considerations in transurethral resection of the prostate. Anesth Intensive Care. 1987;15:203–211.

[42] Swaminathan R, Tormey WP. Fluid absorption during transurethral prostatectomy. Br J Urol. 1981;282:317.

[43] Hawary A, Mukhtar K, Sinclair A, Pearce I. Transurethral resection of the prostate syndrome: almost gone but not forgotten. J Endourol. 2009;23:2013–2020.

[44] Jensen V. The TURP syndrome. Can J Anaesth. 1991;38:90–96.

[45] Hahn RG. The transurethral resection syndrome. Acta Anaesthesiol Scand. 1991; 35:557–1567.

[46] Monk TG, Weldon BC. The renal system and anesthesia for urologic surgery. In: Barash PG, Cullen BF, Stoelting RK, editors. Clinical anesthesia. 4th ed. Philadelphia: Lippincott, Williams & Wilkins; 2001. pp. 105–1033.

[47] Sterns RH, Riggs JE, Schochet Jr SS. Osmotic demyelinization syndrome following correction of hyponatremia. N Engl J Med. 1986;314:1535–1542.

[48] Bevacqua BK. Continuous spinal anaesthesia: What's new and what's not. Best Pract Res Clin Anaesthesiol. 2003;17:393–406.

[49] Malhotra V, Sudheendra V, Diwan S. Anesthesia and the renal and genitourinary systems. In: Miller R, editor. Miller's Anesthesia, vol. 54, 6th ed. Philadelphia: Churchill Livingstone; 2005. pp. 2175–2208.

[50] Rassweiler J, Teber D, Rainer KR, Hofmann R. Complications of transurethral resection of the prostate (TURP)-incidence. Manage Prevent Eur Urol. 2006;50:969–980.

[51] Herkommer K, Hofer C, Gschwend JE, Kron M, Treiber U. Gender and body mass index as risk factors for bladder perforation during primary transurethral resection of bladder tumors. J Urol. 2012;187:1566–1570.

[52] Pahira JJ, Razack AA. In: Hanno PM, Malkowitz SB, Wein AJ, editors. Penn Clinical Manual of Urology, Nephrolithiasis, 3rd ed. New York: McGraw Hill; 2001. pp. 231–252.

[53] Duffty J, Hilditch G. Anaesthesia for urological surgery. Anaesth Intensive Care Med. 2009;10:307–312.

[54] Junghans T, Modersohn D, Dorner F. Systemic evaluation of different approaches for minimizing hemodynamic changes during pneumoperitoneum. Surg Endosc. 2006;20:763–769.

[55] Phong SVN, Kohl LKD. Anaesthesia for robotic-assisted radical prostatectomy: considerations for laparoscopy in the Trendelenburg position. Anaesth Intensive Care. 2007;35(2):281–285.

[56] Badawy M, Beique F, Al-Halal H, et al. Anesthesia considerations for robotic surgery in gynecologic oncology. J Robot Surg. 2011;5(4):235–239.

[57] Samm BJ, Dmochowski RR. Urologic emergencies. Postgrad Med. 1996;100:187–200.

[58] Denny Z, Levvett H. The effect of fluid optimization on outcome following major surgery. Transfus Altern Transfus Med. 2002;4(3):75.

[59] Metzner J, Posner KL, Lam MS, Domino KB. Closed claims' analysis. Best Pract Res Clin Anaesthesiol. 2011;25:263–276.

[60] Welch MB, Brummett CM, Welch TD, et al. Perioperative peripheral nerve injuries: A retrospective study of 380,680 cases during a 10-year period at a single institution. Anesthesiology. 2009;111:490–497.

[61] Weber ED, Colyer MH, Lesser RL, Subramanian PS. Posterior ischemic optic neuropathy after minimally invasive prostatectomy. J Neuroophthalmol. 2007;27:285–287.

[62] Ubee SS, Manikandan R, Athmanathan N, Singh G, Vesey SG. Compartment syndrome in urological practice. BJU Int. 2009;104:577–578.

[63] Cheney FW, Domino KB, Caplan RA, Posner KL. Nerve injury associated with anesthesia: A closed claims analysis. Anesthesiology. 1999;90:1062–1069.

[64] Mizuno J, Yonenaga K, Arita H, Hanaoka K. Right median nerve injury following laparoscopic sigmoidectomy. Masui. 2008;57:752–755.

[65] Pelosi P, Croci M, Calappi E, et al. The prone positioning during general anesthesia minimally affects respiratory mechanics while improving functional residual capacity and increasing oxygen tension. Anesth Analg. 1995;80:955–960.

[66] Warner MA, Martin JT, Schroeder DR, Offord KP, Chute CG. Lower-extremity motor neuropathy associated with surgery performed on patients in a lithotomy position. Anesthesiology. 1994;81:6–12.

[67] Glenn J. Neural damage resulting from dorsal lithotomy positioning. Surg Rounds. 1981;4:42–46.

[68] Kroll DA, Caplan RA, Posner K, Ward RJ, Cheney FW. Nerve injury associated with anesthesia. Anesthesiology. 1990;73:202–207.

[69] Rupp-Montpetit K, Moody ML. Visual loss as a complication of non-ophthalmic surgery: A review of the literature. Insight. 2005;30:10–17.

[70] De Keulenaer BL, De Waele JJ, Powell B, Malbrain ML. What is normal intra-abdominal pressure and how is it affected by positioning, body mass and positive end-expiratory pressure? Intensive Care Med. 2009;35:969–976.

Chapter 4

Obesity and Anesthesia Management

Ismail Demirel, Esef Bolat and Aysun Yıldız Altun

Additional information is available at the end of the chapter

http://dx.doi.org/10.5772/65920

Abstract

The prevalence of obesity is rapidly increasing throughout the world. Correspondingly, anesthetic procedures in obese patients are also increasing due to both treatment of obesity and other surgical problems of obese patients. Anesthesia-related complications are also seen in obese patients than in normal-weighted population. The importance of anesthetic applications in obese patients originates from physiological and pharmacokinetic alterations. Inhalation of these patients via mask or intubation during general anesthesia may be difficult or even impossible. Determination of extubation time after awakening from anesthesia is also a critical decision. Sleep apnea syndrome and postoperative atelectasis are more common in obese patients than in normal-weighted population. Another vital complication that should be emphasized is thromboembolism, whose incidence and severity may be decreased by pharmacological and functional preventive modalities. This patient population has elevated risk of perioperative mortality and morbidity. Prior to any elective surgical procedure, an obese patient should be thoroughly evaluated to check medical conditions that may increase perioperative mortality risk. Since anesthesiologists will gradually encounter more obese patients, they need a better comprehending of the difficulties of obesity during anesthetic procedures and taking more preventive measures for their patients to avoid complications, or rendering them less traumatic, if any.

Keywords: obesity, airway management, drug dosages, perioperative management, postoperative analgesia

1. Introduction

Though obesity is not a newly emerging problem with its epidemic character at both public and individual levels, there has been recent increase in the number of successful surgical interventions with low likelihood of serious morbidity. Body weight of more than 50% of adults in the United States (US) is 20% more than the body weight regarded optimum for the height. The percentage of such adults has increased from 30 to 50% just in 18 years [1].

Overweight has been defined as an excess of total or expected "normal" body weight, including all tissue components (muscle, bone, water, and fat) of body composition. In practice, the terms obesity and overweight are often used interchangeably to refer to excess body fat, but ideally an index of obesity should reflect only excess adipose tissue and be independent of height, body fluids, and muscle, and skeletal mass.

Body mass index (BMI) is now the standard measure for describing different categories of obesity. It must always be remembered that BMI is an indirect measure of obesity since it only considers height and weight, irrespective of the source of any additional weight. BMI is calculated by dividing patient weight (kilograms, kg) by the square of their height (meters, m); BMI = kg/m^2. An increased BMI can be present from any cause of excess weight (body building, ascites, and very large tumor) even in the absence of additional fat. The United States and many countries classify obesity according to BMI, as shown in **Table 1** [2].

BMI	
<20 kg/m^2	Underweight
20–25 kg/m^2	Normal
26–29 kg/m^2	Overweight
30–39 kg/m^2	Obese
≥40 kg/m^2	Morbid obese
≥50 kg/m^2	Super-obese
≥60 kg/m^2	Super-super obese
World Health Organization (WHO) classification: BMI	
30–34.9 kg/m^2	Class I
35–39.9 kg/m^2	Class II
>40 kg/m^2	Class III

Body mass index (BMI) = weight (kilograms, kg) divided by the square of height (meters, m); BMI = Wt (kg)/Ht (m^2).

Table 1. Classification of obesity by body mass index (BMI).

While many obesity complications that pose threat to perioperative period (e.g., airway difficulties or joint problems) may be observed by physical inspection, other complications such as sleep apnea, systemic and pulmonary hypertension, and diabetes mellitus should be comprehensively assessed by careful anamnesis, physical examination, and laboratory tests. Obesity itself, its complications and treatment, is also important for the anesthesiologist. An individual who has 30% excessive weight has a 40% increased mortality risk due to heart disease and a 50% increased mortality risk due to stroke. Hospital costs are also higher in obesity, with increased risk of perioperative morbidity and mortality [3].

Preoperative assessments make perioperative period more efficient, decrease anxiety of both healthcare providers and cared patients, and make patients have realistic expectations which increase satisfaction from pain management and entire perioperative experience. Obesity is a health problem associated with many medical conditions (**Table 2**). Preoperative assessment allows for detection of possible interindividual differences in terms of physiology of airways, pulmonary system, cardiovascular system, metabolic system, and nervous system. Another benefit is the important contribution of anesthesiologists to surgeons in terms of patient's psychological attitude and preparation [4].

Organ system	
Respiratory	Restrictive lung disease, asthma, obstructive sleep apnea (OSA), obesity hyperventilation syndrome (OHS)
Cardiovascular	Hypertension, cardiomyopathy, congestive heart failure, coronary artery disease, peripheral vascular disease, thromboembolism, sudden death
Endocrine/metabolic	Type 2 diabetes mellitus, Cushing's syndrome, hypothyroidism, hyperlipidemia, vitamin deficiencies
Gastrointestinal	Hiatal hernia, inguinal and umbilical hernia, fatty liver, gallbladder stones
Musculoskeletal	Osteoarthritis on weight-bearing joints, low-back pain
Malignancy	Breast, prostate, cervix, uterus, colorectal
Psychiatric	Depression, low self-esteem

Table 2. Obesity-related medical conditions.

2. Preoperative assessment

It is essential to provide a clinical setting that makes obese patients feel comfortable with respect to physical conditions. Outpatient setting or room should be designed according to overweight/obese patients. Primary physicians or surgeons of the patients should not believe mistakenly that they have adequate knowledge about their patients' medical situation. Comorbidities or other accompanying diseases may not frequently be well-documented. Preoperative assessment by anesthesiologist should include the presence of hyperglycemia or type 2 diabetes mellitus, hyperlipidemia, hypertension, coronary artery disease, respiratory problems, liver disease, and obstructive sleep apnea (OSA). As per indicated surgical procedure, impacts of osteoarthritis should be considered regarding positioning of patient especially during elective surgery [5].

An often overlooked, albeit important issue is the evaluation of medical reasons for obesity. Incidence of endocrine disease other than type 2 diabetes mellitus was reported as 47.4% among morbidly obese patients considered for bariatric surgery. Prevalence of hypothyroidism, pituitary diseases, and Cushing's syndrome is shown to be 18.1, 1.9, and 16.3%, respectively. Newly established endocrine diseases are present in 16.3% of all patients [6].

Psychological tests of morbidly obese patients frequently revealed depression, social impairment, and loss of interest in interindividual behaviors. Physicians should be aware of the likelihood of the presence of psychosocial problems in obese patients during the perioperative period [7].

Routine laboratory tests indicated for obese patients are summarized in **Table 3**. If the obese patient had history of bariatric surgery such as gastric bypass or other which represents a potential for malabsorption, a significant protein, vitamin, iron, or calcium deficiency may be present. Therefore, further additional tests are required in such patients to assess metabolic alterations (**Table 4**) [8].

Anesthesiologist should question all current medication of the patient, including over-the-counter and prescribed appetite-stimulating and weight-lowering drugs since most of these agents are associated with serious heart and lung problems and important morbidity and mortality (**Table 5**) [8].

Fasting plasma glucose
Lipid profile
Electrolytes including sodium, potassium, calcium, and phosphorus
Liver function tests including AST, ALT, total, and direct bilirubin
Renal function tests including creatinine level
Complete blood cell count
Ferritin
Vitamin B12
Thyroid stimulating hormone (TSH)
25-Hydroxy vitamin D level
Testosterone level
Electrocardiogram (ECG)
Especially in >55-year-old women and >45-year-old men who has established or suspected heart disease or at higher risk for heart disease
P-A chest X-ray
Especially in >60-year-old patients with established or suspected lung or heart disease
Polysomnography
Other clinically indicated additional tests, such as echocardiography

Table 3. Routine preoperative tests for obese patients.

2.1. Assessment and optimization of airways and pulmonary system

Factors increasing perioperative risks in obese patients in terms of airways and pulmonary system include airway anatomy, rapid desaturation developed during anesthesia induction secondary to reduced functional residual capacity (FRC), tendency to desaturation in supine position, need for induction and recovery in vertical position, tendency to sleep apnea, chronic respiratory insufficiency, pulmonary hypertension, predisposition to deep venous thrombosis and its consequences, and need for active participation to encourage for postoperative mobilization [9].

Test	Month 6	Month 12	Month 18	Month 24	Afterwards
Complete blood count	√	√	√	√	√
Biochemistry profile	√	√	√	√	√
Iron	√	√	√	√	√
Magnesium	√	√	√	√	√
Albumin	√	√		√	√
Vitamin B12	√	√	√	√	√
Vitamin D		√	√	√	√
Other lipid soluble vitamins		√		√	√
Parathyroid hormone	√		√		√
Folate		√		√	√
Bone density		√		√	√
Lipid panel		√			
Uric acid		√			
Vitamin K		√			

Table 4. Preoperative laboratory tests recommended for patients with history of bariatric surgery.

Obesity is a common and important risk factor for obstructive sleep apnea (OSA). A near two-unit increment in BMI raises the probability of OSA by fourfold. While the prevalence of OSA in general population is 2 and 4% in women and men, respectively, it ranges from 3 to 25% and 40 to 78% in morbidly obese women and men, respectively. Sleep apnea in obese patients has usually obstructive character and originated from airway stenosis secondary to excessive amount of peripharyngeal adipose tissue and from reduction of upper airway muscle tonus during rapid eye movement (REM) sleep. BMI, neck diameter, lung function tests (LFT), arterial blood gas measurement during daytime room air, and sleep-related complaints could not adequately predict the presence and severity of OSA in obese patients [10].

Definitive diagnosis of OSA is established by polysomnography, where following criteria should be fulfilled: occurrence of ≥5 apneic events (≥10 s interruption of air flow despite attempting to breath) or ≥15 hypopneic events (>50% reduction of air flow for ≥10 s) per hour during 7-h sleep test. Apneic/hypopneic index (AHI) shows the total number of apneic and/or hypopneic events per slept hour. The severity of OSA is directly correlated with the increase in AHI [11].

The determination of OSA in obese patients has two important implications. First, patients with OSA are more prone to the suppressive effects of hypnotics and opioids on airway muscle tonus and respiration [12]. Postoperative parenteral or neuraxial opioid use may lead to respiratory complications that may result in death or potentially fatal events [13, 14]. Second, OSA complicates laryngoscopy and mask ventilation [15]. Moreover, oxygen stores are decreased due to reduced expiratory reserve volume (ERV) in obese patients [16]. Combination of these factors predispose to serious problems in airways.

Drug	Implications for anesthetic procedures (reported adverse effects)
Diethylpropion	Pulmonary hypertension and psychosis.
Dexfenfluramine	Associated with pulmonary hypertension and cardiac valve disease.
Fenfluramine	Associated with pulmonary hypertension and cardiac valve disease.
Fluoxetine	Selective serotonin reuptake inhibitor. Associated with diarrhea, nausea, headache, and dry mouth. Bradycardia, hemorrhage, convulsion, hyponatremia, hepatotoxicity, and extrapyramidal effects were reported.
Mazindol	Pulmonary hypertension, atrial fibrillation, and syncope episodes were reported.
Metformin	No adverse effect was reported.
Orlistat	Diarrhea and reduced levels of lipid-soluble vitamins were reported.
Phentermine	Association with cardiopulmonary problems could not be excluded.
Phenylpropanolamine	Increases risk of hemorrhagic stroke.
Sibutramine	May lead to mild increases in blood pressure and heart rate. Associated with arrhythmia and hypertension, which is likely to be related to cardiac arrest and stroke.
Diuretics	Hypovolemia, hypokalemia.
Herbal products	
Chitosan	No adverse effect was reported.
Chromium	No adverse effect was reported.
Ephedra	Hypertension, psychiatric symptoms, autonomic dysfunction, gastrointestinal symptoms.
Hydroxycitric acid	No adverse effect was reported.
Pyruvate	Death was reported in a patient with restrictive cardiomyopathy.

Table 5. Weight lowering drugs.

Anamnesis is the easiest way of evaluation of OSA in the preoperative period in patients who did not undergo polysomnography before. Such useful data could be obtained from patient's roommate or sleep partner. Anamnestic data about snoring, interruption of breathing during sleeping (a short-time attempt to inspire after apneic episodes and wheezy breathing or resuscitative nasal breathing), decreased daytime performance, morning headache, and irritability suggest sleep apnea. Systemic hypertension and increased neck diameter (>40–42 cm at cricoid cartilage level) is consistent with probable OSA diagnosis [11, 17]. Other abnormalities of OSA detected during physical examination include somnolence and mask airway and/or intubation difficulties (e.g., Mallampati class III or IV hypognathia, short thyromental distance) [12, 14, 15].

Some obese patients develop chronic daytime hypoventilation, called as obesity-hypoventilation syndrome (OHS) [18]. These patients also have chronic daytime hypoxemia (PO_2 < 65 mmHg), which could be easily detected by pulse oximetry at room air. Permanent hypercapnia ((PCO_2 > 45 mmHg) in the absence of serious obstructive pulmonary disease is pathognomonic for this syndrome in obese patients. These patients usually have advanced obesity (BMI > 40 kg/m^2) and risk of OHS is markedly increased with increasing BMI [19]. Majority of patients with OHS has also OSA; however OHS is not common in OSA patients. Those patients being at the "severe" end of OHS spectrum with cor pulmonale signs and symptoms are called "Pickwickian" [10, 18].

Careful determination of concomitance of obesity and OHS or COPD is important since this combination often leads to chronic daytime hypoxemia, which in turn causes pulmonary hypertension, right ventricular hypertrophy, and/or right ventricular failure. Perioperative morbidity and mortality rates are high in these disorders (Pickwickian), where patients need to undergo many tests to guide for perioperative medical optimization and postoperative care [10, 12, 20].

In perioperative setting, oxygenation is further diminished by reduction in muscular tonus of chest wall and diaphragm following general anesthesia induction and skeletal muscle relaxation. The net effect of this on obesity is the decrease of ERV and FRC by more than 50% and consequent decrease in the number of alveoli making efficient gas exchange, compared to the preinduction phase [21]. In addition, reduction in ERV and FRC increases predisposition to postoperative atelectasis and may inhibit effective clearance of secretions.

Main source of oxygen reserve during apnea is ERV. Therefore, preoxygenation is less effective in obese patients and the time required for hemoglobin desaturation to be reduced to below 90% after apnea is shortened [22]. Obese patients in relaxed condition under anesthesia have increased likelihood of hypoxemic complication due to "reduction in apneic oxygenation reserve" and difficulty of performing positive pressured mask ventilation [15]. In patients considered for bariatric surgery, elective awake tracheal intubation may be the safest approach if there are signs for difficult intubation (e.g., insufficient visualization of posterior pharyngeal wall). Before the induction, after placing a cylinder under the scapula and a support to the occipital region of the patient and asking for full extension at atlanto-occipital joint from the patient may ease awake or conventional laryngoscopy and intubation [23].

A study showed that laryngoscopy was more difficult to perform in obese patients (BMI > 30 kg/m^2) compared to patients with normal BMI [24]. However, authors in another study did not observe any correlation between difficult intubation and BMI, though they found an association between difficult intubation and increased neck diameter (>40–42 cm) or Mallampati score of III or IV [25]. This may be explained by higher probability of incidence of both increased neck diameter and increased Mallampati class in obese patients. Moreover, since obese patients have elevated gastric secretion volume and acidity in the preoperative period, premedication is applied by administration of cimetidine, ranitidine, citric acid, sodium citrate, or metoclopramide. Some investigators suggest this as an indication for awake intubation [26].

2.2. Cardiac assessment

2.2.1. Assessment and prevention of venostasis and thromboembolism

Evaluation of venous system should be prioritized in cardiovascular assessment as implied by mortality data. Venous emboli entered into pulmonary circulation are important causes of pulmonary dysfunction with a 30-day mortality of 1–2%. Majority of 30-day perioperative mortality after bariatric surgery originates from pulmonary embolism (the number of mortality for this reason is ≥ 3 times more than the number of mortality due to anastomosis leakage and consequent sepsis) [27]. Although several agents have been used to diminish the tendency to thrombosis, no consensus has been established. Since low-molecular-weight heparin may limit options for postoperative pain management, preoperative aspirin, and following warfarin (INR 2.0–3.0) may be considered as a reasonable choice. Use of warfarin, a vitamin K antagonist, may elicit some problems during the postoperative period as many patients develop malabsorption of lipids and lipid-soluble substances, including vitamin K after Roux-en-Y gastrojejunostomy (RNYG). Optimizing warfarin dosage may become difficult due to this malabsorption, where daily adjustments are required for at least a couple of weeks [28]. Preoperative exercise, prophylaxis through antithrombotic agents and variceal socks, hematocrit count below the level of polycythemia, increased cardiac output, and early ambulation decrease the risk in this patient group. Therefore, evaluation and prophylaxis including exercise status, pharmacological treatment, absence of symptoms and signs of venous disease and absence of evidence of venous disease, optimal hydration as well as early ambulation should be targeted [29].

2.2.2. Cardiovascular assessment

Cardiac output is expected to increase by 0.01/min for every kilogram of adipose tissue. Consequently, obese patients develop hypertension and associated cardiomegaly and left ventricular failure. To measure blood pressure accurately, an appropriate-sized cuff should be selected, which may not be as easy as it seems. Obesity not only leads to parenteral access difficulty, but also complicates noninvasive blood pressure monitoring. Direct arterial monitoring may be needed for accurate and continuous tracing of blood pressure and frequent arterial blood sampling, based on the extent of cardiopulmonary reserve [30].

Cardiac reserve may be limited in obese patients, where tolerance to hypotension, hypertension, tachycardia, or volume loading-induced stress in preoperative period may be diminished. Most of patients with Pickwickian syndrome also have right-sided heart failure. For this reason, routine preoperative assessment should also include electrocardiogram (ECG) in addition to anamnesis and physical examination featuring drug treatment and cardiopulmonary problems (especially in terms of left or right ventricular hypertrophy, ischemia, and conduction defects). In cases where biventricular failure is severe and not compensated with ≥2 month lasting exercises, measurement of central vascular volume when a large volume of blood loss is expected related to surgery or coagulation status. Physical examination of peripheral venous line may also allow for planning of the possible need for central venous catheter. Some physicians prefer transesophageal echocardiography to assess central volume instead of central venous pressure (CVP) measurement [31]. There are six risk factors to predict perioperative cardiovascular morbidity:

(i) High-risk surgery (e.g., emergent, major thoracic, abdominal, and vascular surgery)

(ii) History of coronary artery disease

(iii) History of congestive heart failure

(iv) History of cerebrovascular disease

(v) Preoperative insulin treatment

(vi) Preoperative plasma creatinine level >2 mg/dL

No additional cardiac tests are required for the elective surgery of patients where these risk factors are absent [32].

2.3. Metabolic assessment

2.3.1. Diabetes mellitus

Although 15% of patients with type I diabetes mellitus has also other comorbid autoimmune diseases such as Graves' disease, Hashimoto's thyroiditis, Addison's disease, and myasthenia gravis, no such an association has been reported in terms of obesity-related diabetes [33].

Current treatment of type II diabetics is initiated with exercise and dietary changes usually. A 5–10 kg weight loss, achieved by a 20% decrease in caloric intake and elevation of daily physical activity to 30 min for a total of 8 weeks often normalize fasting blood glucose levels. Nevertheless, this step is very difficult to achieve for most of patients, and patients will eventually switch to oral hypoglycemic agents, which stimulate secretion of insulin from pancreatic β-cells and improve insulin response of tissues by reversing postbinding defect [34]. Frequently used oral agents include tolazamide, tolbutamide, glyburide, and glipizide, the two latter being sulfonylurea class. Sulfonylureas have more long-lasting glucose-lowering effects (≥24 h) and lower drug-drug interaction potential [35].

By accelerating nonenzymatic glycosylation reactions, higher glucose concentrations lead to the formation of abnormal proteins which decrease flexibility and stretching resistance in wound healing, thereby causing toxic effects. Diminished flexibility may result in stiff joint syndrome and atlanto-occipital joint fixation which could hamper intubation [36].

Anastomosis-related infections are responsible for two-thirds of postoperative complications and about 20% of perioperative mortality in patients undergoing bariatric surgery and constitute number one risk in this patient group. Experimental data show that multiple factors may increase predisposition to infection in patients with glucose intolerance. Many alterations observed in leukocyte functions of hyperglycemic diabetic patients include decreased chemotaxis, impaired phagocytic activity of granulocytes as well as diminished intracellular destruction of pneumococci and staphylococci [37]. Phagocytic functions of granulocytes improve and intracellular killing capacity become near-normal if diabetic patients are aggressively treated, ensuring a blood glucose level <250 mg/dL [38].

2.3.2. *Hypocalcemia*

Inadequate calcium intake is both associated with obesity and hypertension; indeed, normalization of calcium intake could improve both hypertension and eating crises that lead to obesity [39].

2.3.3. *Hyperlipidemia and hypolipidemia*

Dietary control is an important treatment modality in all hyperlipidemia types [40]. Clofibrate and gemfibrozil, which are used for the management of hypertriglyceridemia, may cause myopathy especially in patients with hepatic or renal disease. Clofibrate may also increase the formation of gallbladder stones. Apart from bile acids, cholestyramine also binds to oral anticoagulants, digitalis class agents, and thyroid hormones. Nicotinic acid leads to peripheral vasodilatation, which should be likely to discontinue on the day of surgery. Probucol decreases synthesis of apoprotein A1. Rare malodorous perspiration and/or QT interval prolongation are seen during probucol usage, and sudden death in animals [41].

Hypolipidemia, albeit a rare condition, is associated with neuropathy, anemia, and renal failure. Although anesthesia experience is limited in patients with hypolipidemia, following may be recommended: maintenance of caloric intake and perioperative use of intravenous protein hydrolysates and glucose [42].

2.4. Psychological assessment and psychiatric considerations

Psychological assessment is very important for a successful outcome. Not just a week, but even a whole year following the surgery is not an easy period. Each patient needs to have increased awareness and strong-minded with a dedicated attitude of diarizing his/her diet [7]. Evaluations of anesthesiologist may provide important clues. Patient should be emotionally stable. Anesthesiologist may identify several factors about failure, which include drug abuse, untreated major psychiatric disorders, compulsive eating behavior, fibromyalgia, and chronic fatigue syndrome. Investigation, detection, and sharing of any of these may prevent potential frustration of surgical team and avoid patient getting stressed [43].

2.5. Musculoskeletal system assessment and other considerations for patient positioning

Several other considerations about obesity are also important for anesthesiologist in a prognostic and perioperative manner. Appropriate positioning of the patient, binding of monitoring devices, and performing intravenous access become complicated due to excessive and extensive subcutaneous fat tissue and enlarged extremities. Furthermore, assessment of blood pressure is also more difficult compared to normal-weighted patients (difficulty of selecting appropriate cuff) [44].

Assessment of positioning of obese patients prior to the surgery may abolish some postoperative problems. In a retrospective study, incidence of postoperative ulnar neuropathy was reported to be 29% in patients with BMI > 38 kg/m^2, compared to 1% of the control group [45]. Upper brachial plexus injury may also occur secondary to excessive rotation of the head and cervical vertebra to the contralateral side. Hyperabduction of the arm on the affected side may also lead to lower nerve root injury [46].

2.6. Risk classification

According to ASA Physical Status Classification System; patients with 30 < BMI < 40 are classified as ASA II, patients with a BMI ≥40 are classified as ASA III [47]. Also, for these patients, in 2007, DeMaria et al. suggested a risk stratification tool for bariatric patients. The Obesity Surgery-Mortality Risk Score (OS-MRS) assigns one point to each of five preoperative variables: BMI ≥ 50 kg m^2, male gender, hypertension, pulmonary embolic risk factors, and age ≥45 years. A score of 0–1 is classified as "A," 2–3 as "B," and 4–5 as "C" with associated mortality risks of 0.2, 1.1, and 2.4%, respectively [30]. This system was later validated by a multicenter study of more than 4000 patients [48].

3. Intraoperative management

3.1. Positioning in morbidly obese patients

Prevalence of obesity continues to increase rapidly throughout the world [49]. Therefore, all anesthesiologists should be familiar with this issue not only for obesity surgery, but also for other types of surgery [50]. Inappropriate surgical position may lead to serious physiological problems, and even physical injuries [51, 52]. On the other hand, appropriate position may ease procedures, including especially endotracheal intubation, reduce physiological problems, and minimize neural and soft tissue injury [53].

Operation tables having a carrying capacity of near 400 kg should be used for safe anesthetic and surgical procedures in obese patients. If no special operation table is present, two standard ones having a weight-bearing capacity of 200 kg may be adjoined. Patients should be tightly bound to the table, ensuring supporting of areas prone to pressure by gels and pads. These patients may develop renal failure and potentially fatal complications at even supine positions [54, 55]. In a study, Bostanjian et al. [54] described six patients undergoing bariatric surgery, rhabdomyolysis secondary to gluteal muscle necrosis developed after supine position, where the outcomes were fatal in three of cases.

Head-elevated laryngoscopy position, which is described as the position of head and shoulders above the level of the chest, i.e., above an imaginary horizontal line joining sternal notch and external auditory canal, makes laryngoscopy and intubation easy [56]. The position where the head is lifted 25° and reverse Trendelenburg in induction anesthesia were shown to prolong apnea in obese patients without desaturation [57]. Functional residual capacity (FRC) is severely diminished in the supine position after induction of anesthesia. If the reduction in FRC exceeds closure volume, small airways become also closed, ensuing a ventilation perfusion disturbance [58].

Supine position: Switching from the sitting position to the supine position causes an increase in venous load of the heart in some patients. Reduced diaphragmatic movement by abdominal organs leads to increased respiration work, relative hypoxemia, and marked reduction in lung volumes [59]. Lung volume is further decreased in general anesthesia procedures where muscles are completely paralyzed [60]. Compared to normal-weighed patients, FRC and pulmonary compliance are reduced in the supine position in obese patients, eventually increasing ventilation/perfusion mismatch [59]. All these alterations increase as the body mass index (BMI) is elevated. Induction of the anesthesia is recommended to be performed in the lateral decubitus position to overcome these difficulties [61]. Positive end-expiratory pressure (PEEP) may improve lung functions in mechanically ventilated patients [62]. Prolonged supine position should be avoided in patients with reduced cardiac reserve since venous return to the heart is diminished by increased compression onto the inferior vena cava secondary to abdominal pressure and weight. In such cases, operation table or the patient may be turned to the side so as to decrease aortocaval compression [53, 63].

Trendelenburg position: Patient's head is below the horizontal plane in Trendelenburg position, which may increase operative exposure and decrease bleeding in selected cases. It is less tolerated than that in the supine position. In obese patients who already have limited cardiac reserves, blood in lower extremities is added into central and pulmonary circulation by Trendelenburg position, making it hard to tolerate this position [64]. It should be especially avoided in morbidly obese patients. Further diminished residual capacity and pulmonary compliance in this position also lead to atelectasis and hypoxemia. In addition, endotracheal tube may be displaced depending on the position. In brief, this position is often not preferred in obese patients due to all these factors [53, 63].

Head-upward position: Upper torso of morbidly obese patients should be nearly 35–40° in the sitting position or reverse Trendelenburg position in a way where the operation table allows for adequate ventilation. Such position simplifies mask ventilation and conditions of tracheal intubation.

The combined effect of reverse Trendelenburg position and pneumoperitoneum during laparoscopic gastric bypass surgery decreases femoral blood flow and increases venous stasis, thereby increasing risk of pulmonary embolism. Therefore, prolonged applications of this position should be avoided with altering positions occasional breaks during surgery [65].

Prone position: Prone position was shown to increase oxygenation in normal-weighed patients under anesthesia than that in supine position [66]. As long as the chest and pelvis are supported such adequately that allows for abdominal movements, prone position is usually well-tolerated by obese patients. Cardiovascular functions are preserved when appropriate position and supports are provided. Otherwise, cardiac venous return is diminished by compression onto the inferior vena cava and femoral veins, which in turn leads to decreased volume in the left ventricle, causing hypotension. Prone position in obese patients under anesthesia improves pulmonary functions and increase FRC, pulmonary compliance, and oxygenation [53, 67].

Lateral decubitus position: This position is often tolerated well by obese patients. A decrease in the abdominal fat mass' compression on the abdomen diminishes intraabdominal pressure, which eases diaphragmatic movements during mechanical ventilation. However, maintenance of the same position for a long while may lead to vascular congestion and resulting in hypoventilation in underlying lung [68].

Lithotomy position: This position causes increased venous return and cardiac output, and high risk of thromboembolism secondary to venous stasis after prolonged surgery. Another complication of this position may be the development of compartment syndrome when the lower extremities are inappropriately positioned [53, 69].

3.2. Airway management

Obesity leads to many anatomic alterations in airways. Upper thoracic and lower cervical fat pillows result in a limited range of motion in atlantoaxial joints and cervical vertebra. Excessive tissue folds in the pharynx, short and thickened neck, suprasternal, presternal, and posterior cervical fat tissue, and thick submental fat tissue are formed. All these alterations contribute to potentially difficult airway management, which has been reported as 10.3–20.2% in obese patients compared to 1.5–3.2% of general population [70]. Despite all these anatomical and pathological changes, extent of BMI did not appear to influence difficulty of laryngoscopy. This type of difficulty is rather associated with advanced age, male sex, temporomandibular joint pathology, Mallampati class III and IV, history of obstructive sleep apnea, and abnormal upper teeth [71]. Neck diameter has been defined as the best determinant for intubation difficulty in morbidly obese patients. While the probability of problematic intubation was 5% in patients with a neck diameter of 40 cm, this was found to be 35% in patients with a neck diameter of 60 cm [72]. Increased adipose tissue on pharyngeal walls in obese patients complicates mask ventilation and intubation by leading to alterations in upper airway anatomy. The presence of obstructive sleep apnea is an additional pathology that increases the risk for difficult intubation, hence warranting careful consideration in this patient population [73].

The prevalence of aspiration is low in obese patients, though risk of aspiration-related pulmonary complication is known to be increased in this group [74]. Gastroesophageal reflux that may cause aspiration is common in obese patients. Attention should be paid in patients with history of gastric band application especially in terms of aspiration [64].

Intraoperative ideal ventilation strategies are still contradictory in morbidly obese patients, where diminished lung and thorax compliance is particularly important. The increased amount of thoracic fat tissue is associated with decreased FRC that may be increased by elevation of upper torso though this may not provide an increment as effective as in normal-weighed people [75]. While lung volume is not altered, respiratory load, oxygen consumption, and carbon dioxide synthesis are increased following diminution of lung and thorax compliance, which in turn leads to decreased tolerance to respiratory stress. By causing cyclic alveolar collapse, low FRC and unchanged closure volume induce alveolar injury associated with mechanical ventilation [29]. These patients have predisposition for postoperative atelectasis. An association between the extent of atelectasis and the incidence of postoperative ARDS was also demonstrated [76]. An adequate PEEP administration is important to decrease probability of atelectasis during mechanical ventilation. In obese patients, PEEP provides beneficial effects both on PaO_2 and alveolar-arterial oxygen difference, even these benefits were shown to be more prominent as compared to normal-weighed people [15].

Studies showed that applications of PEEP of 10–15 cm H_2O, lung-protective low tidal volume of 6–8 ml/kg, and pressure limit below 30 cm H_2O proved to be beneficial to obese patients [77]. Combined use of recruitment maneuvers and PEEP revealed better effects on intraoperative oxygenation and compliance compared with PEEP use alone during obesity surgery or in surgical obese patients. A meta-analysis reported that pressure-controlled ventilation and volume-controlled ventilation did not differ in terms of outcomes [78].

3.3. Induction and maintenance

All agents used in anesthesia may also be used in obese patients. However, obesity alters pharmacokinetic parameters depending on the lipid solubility and tissue distribution of the administered anesthetic agent. Nonadipose mass is also increased in obese patients. Drug dosages should be adjusted by considering volume of distribution for loading dose and by considering clearance for maintenance dose. Obese people may highly metabolize lipophilic agents compared to underweight people. Pharmacokinetic studies show that weakly or intermediately lipophilic drugs (e.g., vecuronium) are mainly distributed into nonadipose tissues and the dose needs to be calculated according to the ideal body weight. If the clearance is equal to or less than nonobese patients, the ideal body weight should be taken into account for maintenance dose. If the clearance is increased with obesity, then the total body weight should be considered for maintenance dose.

The ideal body weight is calculated as the sum of 49.9 and 0.89 kg for each cm above the height of 152.4 cm in men, and as the sum of 45.4 and 0.89 kg for each cm above the height of 152.4 cm in women. Agents partially distributed into the adipose tissue have variable pharmacokinetic characteristics; they usually have prolonged and unpredictable effects due to altered volume of distribution and clearance rates, respectively [79].

3.4. Induction agents

3.4.1. Thiopental sodium

Thiopental sodium, a frequently used agent for the induction of general anesthesia, is rapidly distributed to highly perfused organs such as brain, liver, lung, intestines, kidneys, heart, and pancreas after bolus administration into the plasma. Reduced plasma concentration and consequent loss of its effect after a short while depends on its rapid distribution to peripheral tissues. High lipophilicity of thiopental increases its volume of distribution and elimination half-life in obese patients. Due to uptake by fatty tissues, its plasma levels decrease within 10 min after induction and the agent is eliminated via liver. A clearance rate of the drug increases twofold in obese patients compared to patients with normal weight. It is reported that administration of the drug according to nonfat body weight is more reasonable for the purposes of induction anesthesia. Nevertheless, increased cardiac output leads to more rapid distribution of thiopental from its effective compartment into the plasma, hence causing an accelerated awaking in procedures where it is administered as single-dose bolus [5, 11].

3.4.2. Propofol

Although propofol has a high lipophilicity, dose adjustment should be performed according to the total body weight due to its high clearance [80]. Its high lipophilicity and rapid distribution from plasma into peripheral tissue render it as the currently most commonly used induction agent in morbidly obese patients. It could be used safely as total intravenous anesthetic drug. Its short-acting nature after single-dose bolus administration is explained by its redistribution from the compartment it acts on, into the plasma and peripheral tissues. As in thiopental sodium, cardiac output is also an important marker in achieving peak plasma concentrations of this agent. When administered as continuous infusion in obese patients, both its volume of distribution and clearance increases along with increased total body weight [53, 59].

3.4.3. Etomidate

Use of etomidate should be considered in patients with hemodynamic instability. Its use is contradictory due to increased incidence of end-organ dysfunction and in-hospital mortality secondary to adrenal suppressive effects in patients administered etomidate for anesthesia induction. Its induction dose should be adjusted by nonfat body weight due to similar pharmacokinetic and pharmacodynamic properties to propofol and thiopental [53, 59].

3.4.4. Opioids

Opioids were quite commonly used to control sympathetic response to tracheal intubation and surgical stress during induction and maintenance of the anesthesia. These agents effectively block the response to nociceptive stimulation in the perioperative period. Increased cardiac output and alteration in body composition (increased fatty tissue and nonfat body weight) in obese patients may change pharmacokinetic properties of the opioids. Administration of opioids leads to upper airway obstruction, central sleep apnea, obstructive sleep apnea, ataxic respiration, and hypoxemia [53, 59].

Fentanyl, one of the most frequently used opioids in anesthesia, has a significantly higher clearance in obese patients, which exhibits a nonlinear increase with the total body weight [53, 59]. As fentanyl, the onset of action of sufentanyl is 3–5 min. Although it has similar plasma clearance, its volume of distribution and elimination half-life is increased in obese patients compared to normal-weighed patients [53, 59, 81].

Alfentanyl, a derivative of fentanyl, has one-tenth of the potency than that of fentanyl. It is more lipophilic and has lower volume of distribution than that in fentanyl. Increased cardiac output decreases concentration of plasma alfentanyl during early distribution phase [53, 59, 81].

Remifentanyl is an ester opioid, which is rapidly metabolized by tissue and plasma esterases. Its administration by continuous infusion is widely adopted. Effects will terminate within 5–10 min after cessation of the infusion, which should be given adjusted to the ideal body weight. Administration of remifentanyl based on the total body weight in obese patients may cause some adverse effects such as bradycardia, hypotension, and muscle rigidity due to supratherapeutic plasma concentrations [53, 59, 81].

3.5. Inhalation agents

Release of inhalation agents is increased due to high solubility in lipids and excessive fat tissue. Furthermore, obese patients were reported to have slow recovery from anesthesia because of extended release of the inhalation agent from adipose tissue [81, 82]. In fact, this slow recovery not only originates from accumulation in adipose tissue but also from increased sensitivity in central nervous system secondary to decreased blood flow in adipose tissue. On the other hand, duration of recovery after procedures of 2–4 h was reported to be similar between obese and nonobese patients [83]. Recovery time after desflurane and sevoflurane, which have low lipid solubility, is also rapid in obese patients [84]. Torri et al. [85] compared obese and nonobese patients and reported that alveolar and inspiratory sevoflurane concentrations were not much changed, yet exhaling of sevoflurane from alveoli was slower in obese patients.

3.5.1. Isoflurane

Isoflurane is more lipophilic than sevoflurane and desflurane, therefore not commonly used in obese patients. Blood flow is decreased as long as the body weight increases. In clinical practice, impact of body mass index on uptake of isoflurane is not clinically relevant [59, 81].

3.5.2. Sevoflurane

Having low lipophilicity and solubility, sevoflurane is rapidly absorbed and eliminated compared to isoflurane [59, 81].

3.5.3. Desflurane

Desflurane, due to its limited distribution in adipose tissue and least lipophilicity and solubility among available inhalation agents, is recommended in obese patients. Nevertheless, the effect of BMI on the absorption of desflurane is not significant. Recovery and wakening from desflurane than that from isoflurane occur more rapidly in both obese and nonobese patients [59, 81].

3.6. Neuromuscular blockers

Neuromuscular blockers are polar and hydrophilic agents, so they have limited distribution in adipose tissue [86]. Except succinylcholine, administrating doses of neuromuscular blockers are usually calculated according to ideal body weight.

3.6.1. Succinylcholine

This neuromuscular blocker is a short-acting agent with a rapid onset of action. It may be preferred in obese patients in order to provide quick tracheal intubation. Pseudocholinesterase levels and extracellular fluid are elevated in obese patients, which determine the duration of action of succinylcholine and thereby warrant the need for dose adjustment with respect to the total body weight [87].

3.6.2. *Vecuronium*

Vecuronium has a nondepolarizing aminosteroid structure and is mainly eliminated via the liver and gallbladder. Since its duration of action may be prolonged when its dose is calculated according to the total body weight, the dose should be adjusted according to the ideal body weight [88].

3.6.3. *Rocuronium*

Being a weakly lipophilic and quaternary ammonium neuromuscular blocker, it is highly ionized with a limited extracellular distribution. Induction dose of 1.2 mg/kg calculated according to the ideal body weight provides excellent intubation settings within 60 s. Administration dose should be adjusted according to the ideal body weight in order to avoid prolonged drug metabolism [59, 87].

3.7. Reversal of neuromuscular blocking agents

Obese patients have increased risk due to upper airway collapse and use of neuromuscular blockers. Therefore, neuromuscular block should be completely reversed before tracheal intubation. Doses of agents reversing neuromuscular blockers should be calculated according to the total body weight. Rapid and thorough reversal of neuromuscular block is particularly important for early restoration of lung functions during early postoperative period [89].

3.7.1. *Neostigmine*

A delayed time to antagonize neuromuscular block by neostigmine has been reported in obese patients. In the study of Suzuki et al. [90], the time elapsed to make train-of-four ratio as 0.9 increased fourfold than normal to antagonize vecuronium. Block should not be reversed by neostigmine under deep neuromuscular block. Recommended dose for neostigmine is 0.04–0.08 mg/kg, whose total dose should not exceed 5 mg [89, 90].

3.7.2. *Sugammadex*

A modified and most potent derivative of cyclodextrin, sugammadex binds to steroidal muscle relaxants with high affinity. Muscle relaxants are encapsulated within lipophilic cavity. Resultant inclusion complex is excreted through kidneys. Affinity of sugammadex to rocuronium is higher than to either pancuronium or vecuronium. It has no effect on acetylcholine, endogenous steroids, or other muscle relaxing agents. It is not recommended for use in severe renal impairment. In intermediate and deep block, dose calculation is inadequate if done according to the ideal body weight; therefore, the dose needs to be adjusted by the total body weight or ideal body weight plus 40% [89, 91].

3.8. Regional anesthesia

Regional anesthesia may be preferred to avoid potentially difficult airway control or postoperative respiratory complications. Detection of landmarks for central blocks or peripheral nerve blocks is especially very compelling in morbidly obese patients. Seventh cervical vertebra or gluteal fissure may be used to identify midline for central blocks. Distribution of the local anesthetics is hard to estimate due to lipid infiltration into epidural space and increased intraabdominal pressure, in which case 75–80% of normal local anesthetic dose may suffice. Regional block practices are regarded as more difficult in obese patients. In a study of 2020 supraclavicular block applications, success rate in obese patients was 94.3% compared with 97.3% in nonobese patients, which was significantly different [92]. The prospective study by Nielsen et al. [93] with over 9000 regional block procedures showed that the failure rate was 1.62 times higher in obese patients than in nonobese patients. Block procedures may be safely performed under the guidance of ultrasonography in obese patients [93, 94].

4. Postoperative care

Obesity is associated with some problems also during postoperative period. The steps of postoperative care of an obese patient should be carefully assessed before the surgery. Postoperative care should aim to prevent from respiratory dysfunction, hypothermia, hemodynamic instability, thromboembolism, nausea, vomiting, and pain [95, 96].

Monitoring should be continued in the recovery unit, while the patient is in sitting position or the head is upward at 45°. Oxygen support should be maintained until arterial oxygen saturation values return to preoperative levels or the patient becomes completely mobilized. In order to be discharged into the ward, the patient should meet routine criteria for leaving wakening room, no hypopnea or apnea period should occur, and preoperative arterial oxygen saturation values should be reached [96].

The prevalence of myocardial infarction is higher in this group compared to nonobese population. In addition, a new onset of atrial fibrillation may be seen during postoperative period. Close monitoring of these patients should be continued also after the surgery [97, 98].

Although being rare, rhabdomyolysis is a fatal complication in this patient population. Predisposing factors include hypotension, dehydration, immobility, and prolonged surgical interventions. In particular, pain in deep tissues of gluteal region should signal rhabdomyolysis. Creatine kinase levels are elevated in such patients [99].

Obesity is a risk factor for thromboembolism, where prophylaxis is recommended in all surgical interventions, except minor surgery. While oral agents such as rivaroxaban and dabigatran are not recommended for obese patients, low-molecular-weight heparin is recommended for prophylactic purposes [96, 100].

The incidence of postoperative nausea-vomiting is not increased in obese patients, albeit a contradictory issue [101].

An effective postoperative pain management is important to prevent pulmonary complications and provides sufficient respiratory depth. Pain management through intramuscular route is not recommended in obese patients. Opioid-induced upper airway obstruction and respiratory depression are more likely to be seen in obese patients with obstructive sleep apnea. When deciding postoperative analgesia in obese patients, selecting a multimodal analgesia method rather than a unimodal method will provide more effective pain control and avoidance of potential complications [95, 96, 102].

4.1. Intensive care

Obesity was found to be associated with increased need for mechanical ventilation and longer duration of stay with tracheostomy and at intensive care unit. No increase in mortality was shown.

For mechanical ventilation, 5–7 ml/kg of tidal volume calculated according to the ideal body weight is recommended as well as maintaining a peak inspiratory pressure below 35 cm/H_2O [76, 103].

If the obese patient is hemodynamically stable and gastrointestinal system is functional, enteral route is preferred over parenteral route for nutrition. Guideline of Society of Critical Care Medicine and American Society for Parental and Enteral Nutrition reports that hypocaloric nutrition support preserves nitrogen balance and decreases morbidity in obese patients [104].

"Obesity paradox" is defined as the better prognosis of obese patients after acute cardiovascular decompensation despite the established role of the obesity for developing of cardiovascular diseases. Nevertheless, the effects of obesity on critical illness, death, or long-term outcomes are conflicting [105].

Author details

Ismail Demirel*, Esef Bolat and Aysun Yıldız Altun

*Address all correspondence to: ismaildemirel23@gmail.com

Department of Anesthesiology and Reanimation, School of Medicine, Fırat University Elazığ, Turkey

References

[1] Ogden CL, Carroll MD, Kit BK, Flegal KM. Prevalence of childhood and adult obesity in the United States, 2011-2012. JAMA 2014; 311(8): 806–814. doi: 10.1001/jama.2014.732

[2] Buchwald H. Bariatric surgery for morbid obesity: health implications for patients, health professionals, and third party payers. J Am Coll Surg. 2005; 200 (4): 593–604.

[3] Buchwald H. The evolution of metabolic/bariatric surgery. Obes Surg. 2014; 24(8): 1126–1135. doi: 10.1007/s11695-014-1354-3.

[4] Leykin Y, Pellis T, Del Mestro E, Marzano B, Fanti G, Brodsky JB. Anesthetic management of morbidly obese and super-morbidly obese patients undergoing bariatric operations: hospital course and outcomes. Obes Surg. 2006; 16(12): 1563–1569.

[5] Collazo-Clavell ML. Bariatric surgery: important considerations for the primary care provider. Compr Ther. 2008; 34(3–4): 159–165.

[6] Fierabracci P, Pinchera A, Martinelli S, Scartabelli G, Salvetti G, Giannetti M, Pucci A, Galli G, Ricco I, Querci G, Rago T, Di Salvo C, Anselmino M, Vitti P, Santini F. Prevalence of endocrine diseases in morbidly obese patients scheduled for bariatric surgery: beyond diabetes. Obes Surg. 2011; 21(1): 54–60. doi: 10.1007/s11695-010-0297-6.

[7] Zimmerman M, Francione-Witt C, Chelminski I, Young D, Boerescu D, Attiullah N, Pohl D, Roye GD, Harrington DT. Presurgical psychiatric evaluations of candidates for bariatric surgery, part 1: reliability and reasons for and frequency of exclusion. J Clin Psychol. 2007; 68(10): 1557–1562.

[8] Bernstein DP. Cardiovascular physiology. In Morbid Obesity: Peri-operative Management, 2nd edition. Alvarez A, Brodsky JB, Lemmens HJM, Morton J (Eds.), Cambridge: Cambridge University Press, 2010. pp. 1–18.

[9] Vgontzas AN, Tan TL, Bixler EO, Martin LF, Shubert D, Kales A. Sleep apnea and sleep disruption in obese patients. Arch Intern Med. 1994; 154(15): 1705–1711.

[10] Koenig SM. Pulmonary complications of obesity. Am J Med Sci. 2001; 321(4): 249–279.

[11] Sahin M, Bilgen C, Tasbakan MS, Midilli R, Basoglu OK. A clinical prediction formula for apnea-hypopnea index. Int J Otolaryngol. 2014; 2014: 438376. doi: 10.1155/2014/438376.

[12] Dhonneur G, Combes X, Leroux B, Duvaldestin P. Postoperative obstructive apnea. Anesth Analg. 1999; 89(3): 762–767.

[13] Boushra NN. Anaesthetic management of patients with sleep apnoea syndrome. Can J Anaesth. 1996; 43(11): 599–616.

[14] Orlov D, Ankichetty S, Chung F, Brull R. Cardiorespiratory complications of neuraxial opioids in patients with obstructive sleep apnea: a systematic review. J Clin Anesth. 2013; 25(7): 591–599. doi: 10.1016/j.jclinane.2013.02.015

[15] Siyam M, Benhamou D. Difficult endotracheal intubation in patients with sleep apnea syndrome. Anesth Analg. 2002; 95(4): 1098–1102.

[16] Jones RL, Nzekwu MM. The effects of body mass index on lung volumes. Chest. 2006; 130(3): 827–833.

[17] Riley RW, Powell NB, Guilleminault C, Pelayo R, Troell RJ, Li KK. Obstructive sleep apnea surgery: risk management and complications. Otolaryngol Head Neck Surg. 1997; 117(6): 648–652.

[18] Kessler R, Chaouat A, Schinkewitch P, le Faller M, Casel S, Kreiger J, Weitzenblum E. The obesity hypoventilation syndrome revisited. A prospective study of 34 consecutive cases. Chest 2001; 120(2): 369–376.

[19] Kaw R, Hernandez AV, Walker E, Aboussouan L, Mokhlesi B. Determinants of hypercapnia in obese patients with obstructive sleep apnea: a systematic review and meta-analysis of cohort studies. Chest. 2009; 136(3): 787–796. doi: 10.1378/chest.09-0615

[20] Chung SA, Yuan H, Chung F.A systemic review of obstructive sleep apnea and its implications for anesthesiologists. Anesth Analg. 2008 Nov; 107(5): 1543–1563. doi: 10.1213/ane.0b013e318187c83

[21] Pelosi P, Croci M, Ravagnan I, Cerisara M, Vicardi P, Lissoni A, Gattinoni L. Respiratory system mechanics in sedated, paralyzed, morbidly obese patients. J Appl Physiol. 1997; 82(3): 811–818.

[22] Chalhoub V, Yazigi A, Sleilaty G, Haddad F, Noun R, Madi-Jebara S, Yazbeck P. Effect of vital capacity manoeuvres on arterial oxygenation in morbidly obese patients undergoing open bariatric surgery. Eur J Anaesthesiol. 2007 Mar; 24(3): 283–288.

[23] Neligan PJ, Porter S, Max B, Malhotra G, Greenblatt EP, Ochroch EA. Obstructive sleep apnea is not a risk factor for difficult intubation in morbidly obese patients. Anesth Analg. 2009; 109(4): 1182–1186. doi: 10.1213/ane.0b013e3181b12a0c.

[24] Karkouti K, Rose DK, Wigglesworth D, Cohen MM. Predicting difficult intubation: a multivariable analysis. Can J Anaesth. 2000; 47(8): 730–739.

[25] Gonzalez H, Minville V, Delanoue K, Mazerolles M, Concina D, Fourcade O. The importance of increased neck circumference to intubation difficulties in obese patients. Anesth Analg. 2008; 106(4): 1132–1136, doi: 10.1213/ane.0b013e3181679659.

[26] Illing L, Duncan PG, Yip R. Gastroesophageal reflux during anaesthesia. Can J Anaesth. 1992; 39: 466–470.

[27] Klein S, Burke LE, Bray GA, Blair S, Allison DB, Pi-Sunyer X et al. Clinical implications of obesity with specific focus on cardiovascular disease: a statement for professionals from the American Heart Association Council on Nutrition, Physical Activity, and Metabolism: endorsed by the American College of Cardiology Foundation. Circulation 2004; 110(18): 2952–2967.

[28] Arterburn D, Schauer DP, Wise RE, Gersin KS, Fischer DR, Selwyn CA Jr, Erisman A, Tsevat J. Change in predicted 10-year cardiovascular risk following laparoscopic Roux-en-Y gastric bypass surgery. Obes Surg. 2009; 19(2): 184–189. doi: 10.1007/s11695-008-9534-7.

[29] Afolabi BA, Novaro GM, Szomstein S, Rosenthal RJ, Asher CR. Cardiovascular complications of obesity surgery in patients with increased preoperative cardiac risk. Surg Obes Relat Dis. 2009; 5(6): 653–656.

[30] DeMaria EJ, Portenier D, Wolfe L. Obesity surgery mortality risk score: proposal for a clinically useful score to predict mortality risk in patients undergoing gastric bypass. Surg Obes Relat Dis. 2007; 3(2): 134–140.

[31] Kuruba R, Koche LS, Murr MM. Preoperative assessment and perioperative care of patients undergoing bariatric surgery. Med Clin North Am. 2007; 91(3): 339–351, ix.

[32] Poirier P, Alpert MA, Fleisher LA, Thompson PD, Sugerman HJ, Burke LE et al. Cardiovascular evaluation and management of severely obese patients undergoing surgery: a science advisory from the American Heart Association. Circulation. 2009; 120(1): 86–95. doi: 10.1161/CIRCULATIONAHA.109.192575.

[33] Narayan KM, Boyle JP, Thompson TJ, Sorensen SW, Williamson DF. Lifetime risk for diabetes mellitus in the United States. J Am Med Assoc. 2003; 290(14): 1884–1890.

[34] Mayer-Davis EJ, D'Agostino R, Karter AJ, Haffner SM, Rewers MJ, Saad M. et al. Intensity and amount of physical activity in relation to insulin sensitivity. The insulin resistance atherosclerosis study. J Am Med Assoc. 1998; 279(9): 669–674.

[35] Tuomilehto J, Lindstrom J, Eriksson JG, Valle TT, Hämäläinen H, Ilanne-Parikka P. et al. Finnish diabetes prevention study group. Prevention of type 2 diabetes mellitus by changes in lifestyle among subjects with impaired glucose tolerance. N Engl J Med. 2001; 344(18): 1343–1350.

[36] Arguedas JA, Leiva V, Wright JM Blood pressure targets for hypertension in people with diabetes mellitus. Cochrane Database Syst Rev. 2013; 10: CD008277. doi: 10.1002/14651858.CD008277.pub2. Review

[37] Sunahara KK, Sannomiya P, Martins JO. Briefs on insulin and innate immune response. Cell Physiol Biochem. 2012; 29(1–2): 1–8. doi: 10.1159/000337579. Epub 2012 Mar 1.

[38] Osar Z, Samanci T, Demirel GY, Damci T, Ilkova H. Nicotinamide effects oxidative burst activity of neutrophils in patients with poorly controlled type 2 diabetes mellitus. Exp Diabesity Res. 2004; 5(2): 155–162.

[39] Teegarden, D. Calcium intake and reduction in weight or fat mass. J Nutr. 2003; 133(1): 249S–251S.

[40] Sullivan FM, Donnan PT, Love T. Whole population secondary prevention of coronary heart disease in Scotland: the HEARTS database. Stud Health Technol Inform. 2004; 107(Pt 2): 1227–1229.

[41] Rosenbaum M, Leibel RL, Hirsch J. Obesity. N Engl J Med. 1997; 337(6): 396–407.

[42] Emerging Risk Factors Collaboration, Di Angelantonio E, Sarwar N, Perry P, Kaptoge S, Ray KK et al. Major lipids, apolipoproteins, and risk of vascular disease. JAMA. 2009; 302(18): 1993–2000. doi: 10.1001/jama.2009.1619.

[43] Collazo-Clavell ML, Clark MM, McAlpine DE, Jensen MD. Assessment and preparation of patients for bariatric surgery. Mayo Clin Proc. 2006; 81(10 Suppl): S11–7.

[44] Wong AB, Moore MS. Positioning of obese patients in out-of-operating room locations. Anesth Analg. 2007; 104(5): 1306.

[45] Warner MA, Warner ME, Martin JT. Ulnar neuropathy: incidence, outcome, and risk factors in sedated and anesthetized patients. Anesthesiology 1994; 81(6): 1332–1340.

[46] Sawyer RJ, Richmond MN, Hickey JD, Jarratt JA. Peripheral nerve injuries associated with anaesthesia. Anaesthesia 2000; 55(10): 980–991.

[47] https://www.asahq.org/resources/clinical-information/asa-physical-status-classification system

[48] DeMaria EJ, Murr M, Byrne TK, et al. Validation of the obesity surgery mortality risk score in a multicenter study proves it stratifies mortality risk in patients undergoing gastric bypass for morbid obesity. Ann Surg. 2007; 246: 578–82; discussion 83–84.

[49] Kohn M, Booth M. The World Wide epidemic of obesity in adolescents. Adolesc Med. 2003; 14: 1–9.

[50] Dindo D, Muller MK, Weber M, et al. Obesity in general elective surgery. Lancet 2003; 361: 2032–2035.

[51] Buckley FP, Robinson NB, Simonowitz DA, et al. Anaesthesia in the morbidly obese. A comparison of anaesthetic and analgesic regimens for upper abdominal surgery. Anaesthesia 1983; 38: 840–851.

[52] Dominguez-Cherit G, Gonzalez R, et al. Anesthesia for morbidly obese patients. World J Surg. 1998; 22: 969–973.

[53] Cullen A, Ferguson A. Perioperative management of the severely obese patient: a selective pathophysiological. Can J Anaesth. 2012; 59(10): 974–996.

[54] Bostanjian D, Anthone GJ, Hamoui N, Crookes PF. Rhabdomyolysis of gluteal muscles leading to renal failure: a potentially fatal complication of surgery in the morbidly obese. Obes Surg. 2003; 13: 302–305.

[55] Collier B, Goreja MA, Duke BE. Postoperative rhabdomyolysis with bariatric surgery. Obes Surg. 2003; 13: 941–943.

[56] Levitan RM, Kinkle WC, Levin WJ, Everett WW. Laryngeal view during laryngoscopy: a randomized trial comparing cricoid pressure, backward upward-rightward pressure, and bimanual laryngoscopy. Ann Emerg Med. 2006; 47(6): 548–555.

[57] Dixon BJ, Dixon JB, Carden JR, Burn AJ, Schachter LM, Playfair JM, et al. Preoxygenation is more effective in the 25 degrees head-up position than in the supine position in severely obese patients: a randomized controlled study. Anesthesiology 2005; 102(6): 1110–1115.

[58] Salome CM, King GG, Berend N. Physiology of obesity and effects on lung function. J Appl Physiol. 2010; 108(1): 206–211.

[59] Mandal S, Hart N. Respiratory complications of obesity. Clin Med. 2012; 12: 75–78.

[60] Rehder K. Postural changes in respiratory function. Acta Anaesthesiol Scand. 1998; 113: 13–16.

[61] Aono J, Ueda K, Ueda W, et al. Induction of anaesthesia in the lateral decubitus position in morbidly obese patients. Br J Anaesth. 1999; 83(2): 356.

[62] Pelosi P, Ravagnan I, Giurati G, et al. Positive end expiratory pressure improves respiratory function in obese but not in normal subjects during anesthesia and paralysis. Anesthesiology 1999; 91: 1221–1231.

[63] Brodsky JB. Positioning the morbidly obese patient for anesthesia. Obes Surg. 2002; 12(6): 751–758.

[64] Benedik PS, Baun MM, Keus L, Jimenez C, Morice R, Bidani A, Meininger JC. Effects of body position on resting lung volume in overweight and mildly to moderately obese subjects. Respir Care. 2009; 54(3): 334–339.

[65] Nguyen NT, Cronan M, Braley S, et al. Duplex ultrasound assessment of femoral venous flow during laparoscopic and open gastric bypass. Surg Endosc 2003; 17: 285–290.

[66] Mure M, Domino KB, Lindhahl SG, et al. Regional ventilation–perfusion distribution is more uniform in the prone position. J Appl Physiol. 2000; 88: 1076–1083.

[67] Brodsky JB, Oldroyd M, Winfield HN, Kozlowski PM. Morbid obesity and the prone position: a case report. J Clin Anesth. 2001; 13(2): 138–140.

[68] Lohser J, Kulkarni V, Brodsky JB. Anesthesia for thoracic surgery in morbidly obese patients. Curr Opin Anaesthesiol. 2007; 20(1): 10–14.

[69] Domi R, Laho H. Anesthetic challenges in the obese patient. J Anesth. 2012; 26(5): 758–765.

[70] Ogunnaike BO, Jones SB, Jones DB, Provost D, Whitten CW. Anesthetic considerations for bariatric surgery. Anesth Analg. 2002; 95(6): 1793–1805.

[71] Ezri T, Medalion B, Weisenberg M, Szmuk P, Warters RD, Charuzi I. Increased body mass per se is not a predictor of difficult laryngoscopy. Can J Anaesth. 2003; 50(2): 179–183.

[72] Nguyen NT, Ho HS, Fleming NW, Moore P, Lee SJ, Goldman CD, et al. Cardiac function during laparoscopic vs open gastric bypass. Surg Endosc. 2002; 16(1): 78–83.

[73] Lundstrøm LH, Møller AM, Rosenstock C, Astrup G, Wetterslev J. High body mass index is a weak predictor for difficult and failed tracheal intubation: a cohort study of 91,332 consecutive patients scheduled for direct laryngoscopy registered in the Danish Anesthesia Database. Anesthesiology 2009; 110: 266–274.

[74] Engelhardt T, Webster NR. Pulmonary aspiration of gastric contents in anaesthesia. Br J Anaesth. 1999; 83: 453–460.

[75] Sebbane M, El Kamel M, Millot A, Jung B, Lefebvre S, Rubenovitch J, Mercier G, Eledjam JJ, Jaber S, Hayot M. Effect of weight loss on postural changes in pulmonary function in obese subjects: a longitudinal study. Respir Care. 2015 Jul; 60(7): 992–999. doi: 10.4187/respcare.03668. Epub 2015 Apr 7.

[76] Miller PR, Croce MA, Bee TK et al. ARDS after pulmonary contusion: accurate measurement of contusion volume identifies high-risk patients. J Trauma 2001 Aug; 51(2):223–228; discussion 229-30..

[77] Huschak G, Busch T, Kaisers UX. Obesity in anesthesia and intensive care. Best Pract Res Clin Endocrinol Metab. 2013; 27: 247–260.

[78] Aldenkortt M, Lysakowski C, Elia N, Brochard L, Tramer MR. Ventilation strategies in obese patients undergoing surgery: a quantitative systematic review and meta-analysis. Br J Anaesth. 2012; 109(4): 493–502. http://dx.doi.org/10.1093/bja/aes338

[79] Cheymol G. Effects of obesity on pharmacokinetics implications for drug therapy. Clin Pharmacokinet. 2000; 39(3): 215–231.

[80] Ingrande J, Brodsky JB, Lemmens HJM. Lean body weight scalar for the anesthetic induction dose of propofol in morbidly obese subjects. Anesth Analg. 2011; 113: 57–62.

[81] Lemmens HJ. Perioperative pharmacology in morbid obesity. Curr Opin Anaesthesiol. 2010; 23(4): 485–491.

[82] Adams JP, Murphy PG. Obesity in anaesthesia and intensive care. Br J Anaesth. 2000; 85(1): 91–108.

[83] Cork RC, Vaughan RW, Bentley JB. General anesthesia for morbidly obese patients: an examination of postoperative outcomes. Anesthesiology. 1981; 54(4): 310–313.

[84] Arain SR, Barth CD, Shankar H, Ebert TJ. Choice of volatile anesthetic for the morbidly obese patient: sevoflurane or desflurane. J Clin Anesth. 2005; 17(6): 413–419.

[85] Torri G, Casati A, Albertin A, Comotti L, Bignami E, Scarioni M, Paganelli M. Randomized comparison of isoflurane and sevoflurane for laparoscopic gastric banding in morbidly obese patients. J Clin Anesth. 2001; 13(8): 565–570.

[86] Casati A, Putzu M. Anesthesia in the obese patient: pharmacokinetic considerations. J Clin Anesth. 2005; 17(2): 134–145.

[87] Lemmens HJ, Brodsky JB. The dose of succinylcholine in morbid obesity. Anesth Analg. 2006; 102(2): 438–442.

[88] Schwartz AE, Matteo RS, Ornstein E, Halevy JD, Diaz J. Pharmacokinetics and pharmacodynamics of vecuronium in the obese surgical patient. J Anesth Analg. 1992; 74(4): 515–518.

[89] Lemmens HJ, Ingrande J. Pharmacology and obesity. Int Anesthesiol Clin. 2013; 51(3): 52–66.

[90] Suzuki T, Masaki G, Ogawa S. Neostigmine induced reversal of vecuronium in normal weight, overweight and obese female patients. Br J Anaesth. 2006; 97(2): 160–163.

[91] Loupec T, Frasca D, Rousseau N, Faure JP, Mimoz O, Debaene B. Appropriate dosing of sugammadex to reverse deep rocuronium-induced neuromuscular blockade in morbidlyobese patients. Anaesthesia. 2016 Mar; 71(3): 265–272. doi: 10.1111/anae.13344. Epub 2015 Dec 19.

[92] Ingrande J, Brodsky JB, Lemmens HJ. Regional anesthesia and obesity. Curr Opin Anaesthesiol. 2009; 22: 683–686.

[93] Nielsen KC, Guller U, Steele SM, Klein SM, Greengrass RA, Pietrobon R. Influence of obesity on surgical regional anesthesia in the ambulatory setting: an analysis of 9,038 blocks. Anesthesiology. 2005; 102: 181–187.

[94] Schroeder K, Andrei AC, Furlong MJ, Donnelly MJ, Han S, Becker AM. The perioperative effect of increased body mass index on peripheral nerve blockade: an analysis of 528 ultrasound guided interscalene blocks. Rev Bras Anestesiol. 2012; 62: 28–38.

[95] Flores JC. Post-anesthetic care unit management. In Morbid Obesity: Peri-Operative Management. Alvarez AO (Ed). Cambridge: Cambridge University Press, 2004. pp. 339–346.

[96] Nightingale CE, Margarson MP, Shearer E, Redman JW, Lucas DN, Cousins JM. Perioperative management of the obese surgical patient 2015. Anaesthesia 2015; 70(7): 859–876.

[97] Bamgbade OA, Rutter TW, Nafiu OO, Dorje P. Postoperative complications in obese and nonobese patients. World J Surg. 2007; 31, 556–560.

[98] Wang TJ, Parise H, Levy D, D'Agostino RB Sr, Wolf PA, Vasan RS, Benjamin EJ. Obesity and the risk of new-onset atrial fibrillation. JAMA 2004; 292: 2471–2477.

[99] Chakravartty S, Sarma DR, Patel AG. Rhabdomyolysis in bariatric surgery: a systematic review. Obes Surg. 2013; 23(8): 1333–1340.

[100] Stein PD, Beemath A, Olson RE. Obesity as a risk factor in venous thromboembolism. Am J Med. 2005; 118; 978–980.

[101] Kranke P, Apefel CC, Papenfuss T, Rauch S, Lobmann U, Rubsam B, Greim CA, Roewer N. An increased body mass index is no risk factor for postoperative nausea and vomiting. A systematic review and results of original data. Acta Anaesthesiol Scand. 2001; 45(2): 160–166.

[102] Ziemann-Gimmel P, Hensel P, Koppman J, Marema R. Multimodal analgesia reduces narcotic requirements and antiemetic rescue medication in laparoscopic Roux-en-Y gastric bypass surgery. Surg Obes Relat Dis. 2013; 9(6): 975–980.

[103] Ventilation with lower tidal volumes as compared with traditional tidal volumes for acute lung injury and the acute respiratory distress syndrome. The Acute Respiratory Distress Syndrome Network. N Engl J Med. 2000; 342: 1301–1308.

[104] Dickerson RN. Hypocaloric, high-protein nutrition therapy for critically ill patients with obesity. Nutr Clin Pract. 2014; 29: 786–791.

[105] Stamou SC, Nussbaum M, Stiegel RM, Reames MK, Skipper ER, Robicsek F. Effect of body mass index on outcomes after cardiac surgery: is there an obesity paradox? Ann Thorac Surg. 2011 91 (1); 42–47.

Section 4

Complications in Anesthesiology

Chapter 5

Anesthetic Neurotoxicity in Pediatric Patients

Ayse B. Ozer and Sibel Ozcan

Additional information is available at the end of the chapter

http://dx.doi.org/10.5772/65921

Abstract

In recent years, an increasing number of publications have shown the negative effects of anesthetics on the developing brain and have made inquiries about anesthesia for pediatric patients in practice. Anesthesia is applied to millions of children for surgery, imaging, and other invasive procedures; the issue is very serious and concerns. In this chapter, experimental and clinical studies about the issue have been summarized. As a result, anesthetic drugs except alpha-2 adrenergic agonist anesthetic (NMDA antagonist or a GABA agonist) used in pediatric patients (especially if there is no painful situation) have potential neurotoxicity. Particularly, if anesthesia exposure was applied in the fragile period (the first 4 years) and if used at higher concentrations or repeated anesthesia application, adverse effects of anesthesia exposure on the developing brain have been claimed. But, the issue is not fully clarified yet.

Keywords: anesthesia, neurotoxicity, neonatal, developing brain

1. Introduction

Since the beginning of the modern anesthesia (nearly 170 years), millions of people have received inhalation anesthetics, intravenous anesthetics, or a combination in order to create general anesthesia. These drugs have been applied in all age groups, from newborns who may be only a few hours old to geriatric patients. In fact, pediatric patients comprise a significant proportion of the total number of patients treated with general anesthesia, a trend that will continue well into the future.

Pediatric patients are not miniature versions of adult physiology. Pediatric patients differ significantly from adults and among other pediatric patients in anatomical, physiological, and pharmacological characteristics. Many centers have established a separate pediatric anesthesia subspecialty in order to meet the appropriate anesthetic requirements of newborns, premature infants, infants, children, and adolescents. In particular, neonates carry 10 times more mortality and morbidity risk compared to other pediatric age groups. The most common complications in this age group involve the cardiovascular and respiratory system [1]. Holzman [2] noted that the practitioner's experience and the presence of existing respiratory, cardiac, or muscular disease are the key factors that determine the risk of mortality and morbidity. Hemodynamic disturbances due to hypotension, hypertension, tachycardia, bradycardia, asystole, or other arrhythmias arising in the cardiovascular system and respiratory system issues such as hypopnea, apnea, hypoxia, hypocapnia, or hypercapnia can lead to disturbances in microcirculation to the central nervous system (CNS). Although the rate of complications has been reduced through improved understanding of the anatomical, physiological, and pharmacological characteristics of pediatric patients, advances in monitoring methods, and practitioner specialization, the risks are never completely eliminated.

Despite recent advances in the field of pediatric anesthesia, an increasing number of recent reports point to the adverse effects of anesthetics on the developing brain, raising concerns about the application of anesthesia in pediatric patients. As early as 1965, Sir Austin Bradford Hill recognized this issue at a meeting of the Royal Society of Medicine, stating: "How do we determine what are physical, chemical and psychologic hazards of occupation and in particular those that are rare and not easily recognized?" and "… the available human studies … cannot exclude the possibility that the anesthesia- induced neurotoxicity observed in many animal studies may also occur in children" [3]. Although it has been nearly 50 years from that meeting of the Royal Society of Medicine, the short- and long-term effects of anesthesia applications in pediatric patients remain poorly understood. In this chapter, the acute and long-term effects of anesthesia and anesthetics on the developing brain are summarized.

2. Definitions

Neurotoxicity of anesthetic substances on the developing brain is determined by a reduction in neural density and apoptosis in experimental studies and by disturbances in memory, attention, learning, and motor activity in clinical studies [4–6]. Although anesthetic agents used in neonates have known neurotoxic effects, there are valid reasons for using these agents even in vulnerable patients. Because pain itself has a neurotoxic effect, anesthesia-analgesia application in painful conditions may have a net neuroprotective effect [7, 8]. It should also be noted that in cases of hypoxia-ischemia or trauma, administration of anesthetics reduces the infarct volume by reducing the metabolic rate, decreasing intracranial pressure, eliminating free oxygen radicals, and reducing secondary injury [9–11]. Another positive effect is neuroplasticities. These are described as the neurophysical and neurochemical ability to improve compliance against environmental changes and damage when used in depressive disorders and diseases. Neuroplasticity refers to the increase in intercellular connections. Agents that enhance neuroplasticity have raised new hope for the treatment of neurodegenerative diseases [12–14].

3. Other factors that may cause neurotoxicity

Anesthetics are just one of many potential sources of perioperative neurotoxicities. Patient-related factors, such as genetic anomalies, prematurity, sepsis, infection, and vascular diseases, can cause perioperative toxicity. Additionally, hormonal, metabolic, inflammatory, or cardiovascular changes caused by trauma or surgery, hemodynamic disturbances, hypoxia, hypo-/hypercapnia, hypo-/hyperglycemia, electrolyte imbalances, and temperature variations that occur due to anesthesia can also contribute to the development of perioperative neurotoxicity [15–18].

4. Experimental studies

4.1. Inhalation anesthetics

In an experimental study by Shen et al. [4], sevoflurane was applied to neonatal (PND3, PND7, and PND14) and adult rats (PNW7) at concentrations ranging from 1% to 4%. Spatial memory was then assessed in adulthood using the Morris water maze (MWM) test. The PNW7 rats were less sensitive to sevoflurane than neonatal rats. Memory defects were apparent in groups treated with repeated low doses or a single high-dose anesthetic. The authors concluded that neonatal exposure to sevoflurane can result in memory defects in adulthood, with greater deficits seen in animals treated with multiple doses in a short period of time. As a result, the authors recommend that exposure to anesthesia during the neonatal period should be limited in dose and duration. Another study has shown that 4-hour sevoflurane exposure (2.5%) resulted in reduced hippocampal postsynaptic density protein-95 expression without causing any neuronal loss and was associated with learning and memory disturbances [19].

Another experimental study reported that 0.5% minimum alveolar concentration (MAC) sevoflurane applied for 6 hours had no significant effect on apoptosis and S100β levels. Conversely, isoflurane, which is given in the same circumstances, was shown to increase the level of apoptosis and S100β levels [20]. In another study, which evaluated the effects of inhalation anesthetics in neonatal rats, it was demonstrated that sevoflurane, isoflurane, and desflurane increased caspase-3 levels. Interestingly, nitrous oxide application (up to 150% concentration) for 6 hours did not cause neuroapoptosis; however, apoptosis was increased when nitrous oxide was applied with isoflurane [21]. Halothane administered during the prenatal period was associated with neurodegeneration and behavioral changes [22, 23]. Xenon, the currently preferred anesthetic, does not cause neuroapoptosis when used alone; on the contrary, xenon reduced the effects of other inhalation anesthetics when administered first [24].

4.2. Intravenous anesthetics

Zou et al. [5] have examined the effect of ketamine anesthesia duration in newborn rhesus monkeys (PND5, PND6) through silver and Fluoro-Jade C stains and caspase-3 immunostain. Three hours exposure to ketamine did not produce any significant histochemical change, whereas profound brain cell death was observed in the frontal cortex among subjects that were under the effect of ketamine for 9 or 24 hours. In cell culture study of Bosnjak et al. [25], they demonstrated that ketamine decreases neuronal viability time and dose dependently, leads to neuronal ultrastructural abnormalities, causes depolarization of mitochondrial membrane potential, induces apoptotic pathway, causes cytochrome c release from mitochondria into cytosol, and induces free oxygen radical production.

Yu et al. examined neuroapoptosis and long-term behavioral changes in PND7 rats that were given single and repetitive doses of propofol. Their findings included reduction in neuron density, morphological changes in pyramidal cells, apoptosis, and suppressed release of excitatory neurotransmitters. Additionally, these effects were more pronounced among the group that was subject to repeated doses of propofol [26].

Benzodiazepines (clonazepam, diazepam, and midazolam), which are intravenous anesthetics, have controversial effects on apoptosis; however, barbiturates (pentobarbital, phenobarbital) clearly increase apoptosis. The few studies that have examined the effects of sodium thiopental reported that exposure did not result in increased apoptosis [27–33]. Thompson [34] has suggested high-dose narcotic anesthetic for neonatal and infant. But, fetal and neonatal chronic exposure to opioids has been associated with neuronal changes. Although opioid-based anesthesia and opioids coadministered with inhalation anesthetics have been shown to reduce apoptosis, safety has not been demonstrated with these preparations [35, 36]. However, these studies are controversial and their safety has been in question. Another study has demonstrated that dexmedetomidine, the current intravenous anesthetic, reduces prenatal toxicity caused by propofol [37].

5. Pathogenesis

The molecular pathogenesis of anesthesia-induced neurotoxicity has also been investigated in experimental studies.

Neonates are born with approximately 100 billion neurons, and the number of neurons does not increase over time. The neonatal brains weigh approximately 300–400 g. Increased myelination, synapse formation, neuron maturation, and proliferation of glial cells increase the weight of the brain to 1100 g at 3 years of age and 1300–1400 g at adulthood. A newborn infant has approximately 50 trillion synapses, increasing to 1000 trillion within the first year of life and decreasing to 500 trillion in adulthood. Critical periods for brain development are the intrauterine period, the first 3 years of life and puberty [38–40].

Thus, brain maturation is not complete at birth, and there is a heterogeneous maturation process in the brain following birth. Maturation is particularly slow in the cortex and in the limbic system [38–40]. Alteration of neurotransmission in the immature brain due to anesthesia exposure may lead to future impairments.

Synaptogenesis has been defined as the most important period of brain development, also described as the "fragile period" or "critical period." Synaptogenesis consists of five phases. The greatest leap in synapse formation occurs in phase 3, which is sometimes referred to as the "big bang." Phase 3 corresponds to the neonatal period. Following phase 3, synaptogenesis continues with the same speed during phase 4. This phase is referred to as the plateau phase, corresponding to infancy and adolescence. During phase 5, which occurs during adulthood, synaptogenesis continues, but it is limited and localized [41]. The initiation, duration, and end of these critical periods (phase 3 and phase 4) are controlled by multiple genetic and epigenetic mechanisms. The brain's sensitivity to environmental stimuli is at maximum during the neonatal and infancy period when synaptogenesis is also maximized [41].

Anesthetics elicit their effects by enhancing the activity of major inhibitory neurotransmitters gamma-aminobutyric acid (GABA) and glycine or antagonizing the N-methyl-D-aspartate (NMDA) receptors of the major excitatory neurotransmitter glutamate. During brain development, GABA facilitates cell proliferation, neuroblast migration, and dendritic maturation, and unlike in adults, it acts as an excitatory neurotransmitter during infancy rather than an inhibitory neurotransmitter [42, 43]. This is because these two mediators increase the permeability of the cell membrane to chloride ions through intrinsic chloride-conducting ion pores. After the permeability of the GABA, ligand-gated ion channel to chloride is increased, KCC2 K+/Cl-2 cotransporter aids in influx of chloride ion. Thus, the neuron is hyperpolarized and its activity is suppressed. However, because KCC2 expression is low during the early period of development, the chloride action potential is reversed by $GABA_A$ and glycine receptor activity, leading to neuronal depolarization and increased permeability to chloride. Clinical studies have shown that sevoflurane, isoflurane, and propofol cause excitability in electroencephalogram in neonates [44–46]. The major excitatory neurotransmitters glutamate and aspartate are present in the brain at very high concentrations (glutamate 10 mmol/L and aspartate 4 mmol/L). Glutamate and aspartate direct synaptic signaling at nerve terminals and control ion intake to neurons. They have been found to influence synaptogenesis, neuronal plasticity, learning, and memory [47–49]. Although the excitatory neurotransmitters are normally responsible for nerve conduction, they are also potential sources of neurotoxicity. An abnormal decrease in glutamate may disturb normal excitation, and abnormal increases may cause excitotoxicity and cell death by disturbing calcium homeostasis. Glutamate and similar amino acids have been shown to cause acute swelling in the neuron body, dendrites, and glia and also promote neuronal degeneration over extended periods of time. For this reason, there is a delicate mechanism acting in normal conditions to regulate glutamate levels in the synaptic gap involving reuptake of excess glutamate from the synaptic gap through receptors present in presynaptic end of nerve terminal and glial cells. Although glutamate is a strong and rapid-acting toxin under physiological conditions, this mechanism ensures that even direct application to the brain does not cause damage [47]. Nevertheless, pathological conditions that result in insufficiency of this system or cause release of large amounts of glutamate would lead to neuronal loss. For these reasons, anesthesia applications are believed to disrupt the balance between excitatory and inhibitory neurotransmission and thus cause neuronal injury [47–49].

Regarding neuronal viability and development, one of the most studied neurotropins in neonatal subjects is brain-derived neurotrophic factor (BDNF). Mature BDNF is formed by destruction of proBDNF in the synaptic gap by the action of plasmin. Mature BDNF binds to the TrkB receptors present on the postsynaptic membrane and enhances viability of the target cell. However, in conditions where plasmin release is reduced or blocked, such as when anesthesia is applied, proBDNF cannot be converted to the mature form, and it stimulates p75NTR instead of the TrkB receptor. Activation of p75NTR receptor, also called the "death receptor," leads to actin depolymerization and apoptosis. Head et al. [50] demonstrated that isoflurane causes apoptosis in the neonatal mice brain through this pathway.

Apoptosis is a programmed cell death that can occur in both physiological and pathological conditions. Apoptosis is physiologically present in the developing brain, occurring at a rate of approximately 1%. However, apoptosis that occurs following pathological processes like hypoxia and ischemia is typically problematic. Several experimental studies have shown that apoptosis is increased following anesthesia exposure. However, it is not possible to conduct such studies in humans. Therefore, it is difficult to estimate the rate of apoptosis following anesthesia exposure in humans to what extent this apoptosis affects maturation of the developing brain. Experimental studies have shown that anesthesia induces apoptosis via intrinsic and extrinsic pathways. Anesthesia application causes leakage of cytochrome c and translocation of Bax protein to the mitochondria, leading to activation of the apaf-1 and caspase pathways, respectively. This in turn results in lipid peroxidation via release of free oxygen radicals. Apoptosis occurs not only in intrinsic pathway but also in extrinsic pathway which activates Fas protein [51–53].

There are three publications that demonstrate the relationship between microRNA and anesthetic-induced developmental neurotoxicity; according to these publications, while propofol downregulates microRNA-21, ketamine upregulates microRNA-34a, microRNA-34c, and microRNA-124 and downregulates microRNA-137 [54–56].

In cell culture models, it has been demonstrated that neuron development is highly dependent on the actin cytoskeleton, and anesthetics are dangerous for actin regulation [57–59].

Tau protein hyperphosphorylation at serine 404 demonstrates neurodegeneration and is induced by ketamine. Therefore, microtubules are disrupted and damaged [60].

Translocator protein (TSPO, 18 kDa) is a biomarker that could be used for evaluation of reactive gliosis and microglia activity and has the potential for use in noninvasive imaging using positron emission tomography and single photon emission computed tomography [61]. The relationship between anesthesia-associated neurotoxicity and DNA methylation and gene expression has been investigated [62].

Treatment strategies to reduce neurodegeneration induced by anesthetics have also been widely investigated. Lithium, melatonin, estradiol, pilocarpine, dexmedetomidine, xenon, erythropoietin, L-carnitine, hydrogen gas, and pramipexole are among the leading candidates for this emerging therapy [63, 64].

6. Clinical studies

Although many experimental studies have been conducted, this alone is not sufficient evidence to conclude that general anesthetics have a neurotoxic effect on the developing human brain. Even within mammals, species vary widely in the rate and timing of brain development. Total maturation of the brain takes only a few weeks in the rat, while maturation of the human brain occurs over many years. In addition, the dose and duration of anesthetics used in experimental models is not directly proportional to the procedures used in patients. In some cases, experimental doses may be as much as 20 times the standard clinical dose. Adjusted for the life span of a rat, 6 hours of anesthesia may correspond to 1 month of a human life span. Again, some observations from these studies, such as lactic acidosis, hypercarbia, and hypoglycemia, have mostly been ignored. Learning ability is also disturbed in subjects that are fasted for the duration of the anesthesia treatment [43, 65, 66].

In one retrospective birth cohort study that used New York State Medicaid data collected between the years 1999 and 2002, 383 children who underwent inguinal hernia repair with anesthesia before the age of 3 were evaluated along with 5050 children who did not undergo an operation. Hazard ratios regarding behavioral and developmental disorders were reported to be 2.3 with exposure to anesthesia, 1.0 for age, 2.7 for gender, 1.2 for race, and 1.6 for birth complications [6]. Considering that elective surgeries can be postponed, exposure to anesthesia is an avoidable risk for most infants.

In another report, patients that had been overexposed to anesthesia had more learning difficulties than those who were treated with appropriate doses. The risk of learning difficulties was progressively increased with repeated exposure to anesthesia [67, 68]. The effects of anesthesia used during cesarean procedures were examined in children. Infants born under regional anesthesia exhibited fewer learning difficulties in the later stages of their life [69, 70].

One retrospective study examined 10,450 siblings born between the years 1999 and 2005 and evaluated developmental and behavioral disorders among those who did and did not receive anesthesia prior to the age of 3. The incidence of developmental and behavioral disorder was 128.2/1000/year among those who were exposed to anesthesia and 56.3/1000/year among those who were not exposed to anesthesia. Therefore, behavioral disorders were 60% more frequent among those who received anesthesia in comparison to those who did not. The estimated hazard ratio for developmental and behavioral disorders was 1:1 for those who received anesthesia once before the age of 3, 2:9 for those exposed twice, and 4 for those who had been exposed to anesthesia three or more times [71].

Meyer et al. observed development of convulsion with similar clinical characteristics in three infants under the age of 2 months, occurring after 23–30 hours of anesthesia induced and maintained using propofol. They reported that the seizures did not recur; however, two infants had progressive microcephaly and cognitive and behavioral disorder. Magnetic resonance imaging also showed white matter abnormalities [72]. The manufacturer of propofol does not recommend the use of propofol as a general anesthetic agent for children under the age of 3 [73].

Clinical studies in the literature are often retrospective, and even strong correlations are not evidence of causality. Therefore, the Mayo Anesthesia Safety in Kids (MASK) study was launched by Mayo Clinic at the suggestion of the FDA to evaluate neurotoxicity in children exposed to anesthesia. The study included children born in Olmsted County between 1997 and 2007 and who still lived there when they reached 8 years old. Those who received general anesthesia before the age of 3 were excluded from the study. Children classified as having single, multiple, or no anesthesia exposure were evaluated between the years 2007 and 2016, when they were at the age of 8–12 or 15–19 with a single session that lasted for 4 hours using the National Center for Toxicological Research-Operant Test Battery (NCTR-OTB). The NCTR-OTB test evaluates processing speed; cognitive/intellectual memory; attention, language, motor and visual-spatial, and cognitive processing; and executive functions [74].

The Pediatric Anesthesia and Neurodevelopmental Assessment (PANDA), which was conducted by the University of Columbia and followed sibling pairs under the age of 3 who underwent inguinal operation up to the age of 8–15, published four symposiums in 2-year interval. The first meeting in 2008 established the goals of the study. The second meeting in 2010 was interdisciplinary. The third meeting in 2012 was attended by different disciplines, parents, clinicians, FDA workers, and patient's rights advocates. In this meeting, attendees agreed to collaborate on advanced preclinical, clinical, and translational studies [75, 76]. Additionally in 2012, pediatric anesthesiologists and pediatric surgeons met to discuss the neurotoxicity risk of some elective procedures and anesthesia applications performed in children and specifically to discuss questions and concerns of parents. Meeting attendees, including pediatric general surgeons, urologists, plastic surgeons, and ophthalmologists, reviewed inguinal hernia, hypospadias-undescended testis, cleft lip, craniosynostosis, cataracts, and strabismus applications in early childhood. They emphasized that the amount of volatile anesthetics and sedation levels could be reduced by using balanced anesthesia methods, regional anesthesia methods, and the use of opioid and non-opioid analgesics, but the group was unable to reach a consensus on best practices [77]. At the 2014 meeting, the existing clinical studies, General Anesthesia Study (GAS), MASK, and PANDA, were evaluated, and Strategies for Mitigating Anesthesia-Related neuroToxicity in Tots (SmartTots) was presented along with the future targets of this organization. SmartTots is a public-private partnership that investigates the effects of anesthetic agents on neural development in infants and children. All panelists evaluated their anesthesia and clinical practices with the following questions [78, 79]:

- What does anesthesia mean to my patients?

- What does anesthesia mean to my practice now?

Ordering imaging studies with sedation/anesthesia.

A child requiring multiple procedures under GA overtime.

A child requiring multiple procedures from different subspecialties at the same time.

- If anesthesia affects neurodevelopment:

How will I discuss this with the parents?

Will I change my practice and how?

The 2014 report indicated that the collected data was insufficient to draw any conclusions. However, it stated 2 years later that the results would be considered as a public health problem, leading to greater awareness [78]. On the other hand, the General Anesthesia Study

(GAS), which is currently ongoing and only investigates causality, investigated cases that were less than 60 weeks from conception and greater than 26 weeks gestational age and had undergone inguinal hernia operations with sevoflurane-based general anesthesia or awake-regional anesthesia. This study was conducted in 28 hospitals from Australia, Italy, the USA, the UK, and Canada. No opioids or nitrous oxide was used. Regional techniques and intravenous acetaminophen were used for postoperative analgesia. Protocols were applied in order to prevent development of adverse states that would contribute in neurotoxicity, such as hypoglycemia, hypotension, and hypoxia. Children were assessed using the composite cognitive score of the Bayley Scales of Infant and Toddler Development III test at the age of 2 and with the Wechsler Preschool and Primary Scale of Intelligence Third Edition (WPPSI-III) Full Scale Intelligence Quotient score at the age of 5. During 2007–2013, 363 infants were enrolled in the awake-regional group, and 359 infants were enrolled in the general anesthesia group. According to the study results, the median general anesthesia duration was 54 minutes. No significant difference was found between the groups regarding cognitive composite score at 2 years of age. This study provides strong evidence that sevoflurane anesthesia lasting <1 hour in infants does not produce more severe neurotoxicity at the second year of age than awake-regional treatment. Nonetheless, the primary outcome of this study is the evaluation of neurodevelopmental state at 5 years of age, and this result has not been published yet. It was also reported in this study that early-period apnea development (<30 minutes) was less frequent in the regional anesthesia group [80].

Other discussed topics are applied anesthesia techniques to mothers during childbirth. Flick et al. determined that neuraxial labor analgesia for vaginal delivery did not cause learning disabilities in childhood [69, 70].

Another topic of discussion was how parents should be informed and the need to establish a protocol. However, since it was not possible to reach a consensus based on the current data, it was concluded that it would not be appropriate to inform parents and establish a protocol yet [81].

Author details

Ayse B. Ozer* and Sibel Ozcan

*Address all correspondence to: abelinozer@gmail.com

Faculty of Medicine, Department of Anesthesiology Intensive Care, Firat University, Elazig, Turkey

References

[1] Cohen MM, Cameron CB, Duncan PG: Pediatric anesthesia morbidity and mortality in the perioperative period. Anesth Analg 1990; **70**:160–167.

[2] Holzman RS:. Morbidity and mortality in pediatric anesthesia. Pediatr Clin North Am. 1994;**41**:239–256.

[3] Flick RP, Warner DO: a users' guide to interpreting observational studies of pediatric anesthetic neurotoxicity. The lessons of sir Bradford Hill. Anesthesiology 2012; **117**:459–462

[4] Shen X, Liu Y, Xu S, Zhao Q, Guo X, Shen R, Wang F: Early life exposure to sevoflurane impairs adulthood spatial memory in the rat. NeuroToxicology 2013;**39**:45–56

[5] Zou X, Patterson TA, Divine RL, Sadovova N, Zhang X, Hanig JP, et al: Prolonged exposure to ketamine increases neurodegeneration in the developing monkey brain. Int J Dev Neurosci 2009;**27**:727–731

[6] DiMaggio, Sun LS, Kakavouli A, Byrne MW, Li G: A retrospective cohort study of the association of anesthesia and hernia repair surgery with behavioral and developmental disorders in young children. J Neurosurg Anesthesiol 2009;**21**:286–291

[7] Sanders RD, Ma D, Brooks P, Maze M: Balancing paediatric anaesthesia: preclinical insights into analgesia, hypnosis, neuroprotection, and neurotoxicity. Br J Anaesth 2008;**101**:597–609.

[8] Hays SR, Deshpande JK. Neurotoxicity of anesthesia on developing brain. In: Baheti DK, Dhayagude SH, Deshpande JK, Menon R, editors. World clinics, anesthesia, critical care, pain, pediatric anesthesia-II. 2nd ed. New Delhi: Jaypee Brothers Medical Publishers Ltd;. 2015. p. 117–143

[9] Tawfeeq NA, Halawani MM, Al-Faridi K, Aal-Shaya WA, Taha WS: Traumatic brain injury: neuroprotective anaesthetic techniques, an update. Injury 2009;**40**:S75–S81.

[10] Burchell SR, Dixon BJ, Tang J, Zhang JH: Isoflurane provides neuroprotection in neonatal hypoxic ischemic brain injury. J Investig Med. 2013;**61**:1078–1083.

[11] Stocchetti N, Taccone FS, Citerio G, Pepe PE, Le Roux PD, Oddo M, et al: Neuroprotection in acute brain injury: an up-to-date review. Crit Care 2015;**19**:186.

[12] Kays JL, Hurley RA, Taber KH: The dynamic brain: neuroplasticity and mental health. J Neuropsychiatry Clin Neurosci. 2012;**24**:118–124.

[13] Zheng Z, Xu F: Neuroplasticity may play a role in inter-individual difference among neuropsychiatric disease treatment efficacy. Dev Psychobiol. 2012;**54**:369–371.

[14] Cramer SC, Sur M, Dobkin BH, O'Brien C, Sanger TD, Trojanowski JQ, et al: Harnessing neuroplasticity for clinical applications. Brain. 2011;**134**:1591–1609.

[15] Soriano SG, Anand KJ: Anesthetics and brain toxicity. Curr Opin Anaesthesiol 2005;**18**:293–297.

[16] Taylor J: Anaesthesia-induced developmental neurotoxicity. South Afr J Anaesth Analg 2012;**18**:242–247.

[17] Davidson AJ: Anesthesia and neurotoxicity to the developing brain: the clinical relevance. Pediatr Anesth 2011;**21**:716–721

[18] Wise-Faberowski L, Loepke A: Anesthesia during surgical repair for congenital heart disease and the developing brain: neurotoxic or neuroprotective? Pediatr Anesth 2011;**21**:554–559

[19] Wang SQ, Fang F, Xue ZG, Cang J, Zhang XG: Neonatal sevoflurane anesthesia induces long-term memory impairment and decreases hippocampal PSD-95 expression without neuronal loss. Eur Rev Med Pharmacol Sci 2013;**17**:941–950

[20] Liang G, Ward C, Peng J, Zhao Y, Huang B, Wei H: Isoflurane causes greater neurodegeneration than an equivalent exposure of sevoflurane in the developing brain of neonatal mice. Anesthesiology. 2010;**112**:1325–1334

[21] Istaphanous GK, Howard J, Nan X, Hughes EA, McCann JC, McAuliffe JJ, et al: Comparison of the neuroapoptotic properties of equipotent anesthetic concentrations of desflurane, isoflurane, or sevoflurane in neonatal mice. Anesthesiology. 2011;**114**:578–587

[22] Chalon J, Tang CK, Ramanathan S, Eisner M, Katz R, Turndorf H. Exposure to halothane and enflurane affects learning function of murine progeny. Anesth Analg 1981;**60**:794–797

[23] Quimby KL, Aschkenase LJ, Bowman RE, Katz J, Chang LW: Enduring learning deficits and cerebral synaptic malformation from exposure to 10 parts of halothane per million. Science 1974;**185**:625–627

[24] Cattano D, Williamson P, Fukui K, Avidan M, Evers AS, Olney JW, et al: Potential of xenon to induce or to protect against neuroapoptosis in the developing Mouse brain. Can J Anaesth 2008;**55**:429–436.

[25] Bosnjak ZJ, Yan Y, Canfield S, Muravyeva MY, Kikuchi C, Wells CW, et al: Ketamine induces toxicity in human neurons differentiated from embryonic stem cells via mitochondrial apoptosis pathway. Curr Drug Saf. 2012;**7**:106–119.

[26] Yu D, Jiang Y, Gao J, Liu B, Chen P: Repeated exposure to propofol potentiates neuroapoptosis and long-term behavioral deficits in neonatal rats. Neurosci Lett. 2013;**534**:41–46.

[27] Ikonomidou C, Bittigau P, Ishimaru MJ, Wozniak DF, Koch C, Genz K, et al:. Ethanol-induced apoptotic neurodegeneration and fetal alcohol syndrome. Science 2000;**287**:1056–1060.

[28] Bittigau P, Sifringer M, Genz K, Reith E, Pospischil D, Govindarajalu S, et al: Antiepileptic drugs and apoptotic neurodegeneration in the developing brain. Proc Natl Acad Sci U S A 2002;**99**:15089–15094.

[29] Stefovska VG, Uckermann O, Czuczwar M, Smitka M, Czuczwar P, Kis J, et al: Sedative and anticonvulsant drugs suppress postnatal neurogenesis. Ann Neurol 2008;**64**:434–445.

[30] Young C, Jevtovic-Todorovic V, Qin YQ, Tenkova T, Wang H, Labruyere J, et al: Potential of ketamine and midazolam, individually or in combination, to induce apoptotic neurodegeneration in the infant mouse brain. Br J Pharmacol 2005;**146**:189–197.

[31] Jevtovic-Todorovic V, Hartman RE, Izumi Y, Benshoff ND, Dikranian K, Zorumski CF, et al: Early exposure to common anesthetic agents causes widespread neurodegeneration in the developing rat brain and persistent learning deficits. J Neurosci 2003;**23**:876–882.

[32] Mintz CD, Barrett KM, Smith SC, Benson DL, Harrison NL: Anesthetics interfere with axon guidance in developing mouse neocortical neurons in vitro via a gamma-aminobutyric acid type a receptor mechanism. Anesthesiology 2013;**118**:825–833.

[33] Fredriksson A, Ponten E, Gordh T, Eriksson P: Neonatal exposure to a combination of N-methyl-D- aspartate and gamma-aminobutyric acid type a receptor anesthetic agents potentiates apoptotic neurodegeneration and persistent behavioral deficits. Anesthesiology 2007;**107**:427–436.

[34] Thompson ME: Preventing neurotoxicity: don't forget high-dose narcotic anesthetic. Pediatr Anesth 2014;**24**:1109–1114

[35] Niu L, Cao B, Zhu H, Mei B, Wang M, Yang Y, et al: Impaired in vivo synaptic plasticity in dentate gyrus and spatial memory in juvenile rats induced by prenatal morphine exposure. Hippocampus. 2009;**19**:649–657

[36] De Graaf J, van Lingen RA, Valkenburg AJ, Weisglas-Kuperus N, Groot Jebbink L, Wijnberg-Williams B, et al: Does neonatal morphine use affect neuropsychological outcomes at 8 to 9 years of age? Pain. 2013;**154**:449–458.

[37] Li J, Xiong M, Nadavaluru PR, Zuo W, Ye JH, Eloy JD, et al: Dexmedetomidine attenuates neurotoxicity induced by prenatal propofol exposure. J Neurosurg Anesthesiol. 2016;**28**:51–64.

[38] Graham J. Forstadt LA. Bulletin#4356, Children and brain development: what we know about how children learn. Available from: https://extension.umaine.edu/publications/4356e/

[39] Stages of brain development. Available from: http://www.brainwave.org.nz/wp-content/uploads/2012/05/stages-in-brain-dev.pdf

[40] Early childhood brain development sets the stage for learning throughout life, experts say. Available from: http://www.cleveland.com/healthfit/index.ssf/2015/10/brain_development_is_an_intricate_choreographed_dance_with_many_opportunities_for_missteps_photos.html.

[41] Bourgeois JP. Neonatal synaptic big bang. In: Lagercrantz H, Hanson MA, Ment LR, Donald MP, editors. The newborn brain: neuroscience and clinical applications. 2nd ed. NewYork: Cambridge University Press; 2010. p. 71–85

[42] de Lima AD, Opitz T, Voigt T: Irreversible loss of a subpopulation of cortical interneurons in the absence of glutamatergic network activity. Eur J Neurosci 2004; **19**:2931–2943.

[43] Yu D, Liu B: Developmental anesthetic neurotoxicity: from animals to humans? J Anesth 2013;**27**:750–756

[44] Veyckemans F: Excitation phenomena during sevoflurane anesthesia in children. Curr Opin Anesthesiol 2001;**14**:339–343

[45] Harrison JL: Postoperative seizures after isoflurane anesthesia. Anesth Analg 1986;**65**:1235–1236

[46] Zeiler SR, Kaplan PW: Propofol withdrawal seizures (or not). Seizure 2008;**17**:665–667.

[47] Beal MF: Does impairment of energy metabolism result in excitotoxic neuronal death in neurodegenerative illnesses. Ann Neurol 1992;**31**:119–130

[48] Choi DW: Calcium-mediated neurotoxicity: relationship to specific channel types and role in ischemic damage Trends Neurosci. 1988;**11**:465–469

[49] Choi DW: Glutamate neurotoxicity and diseases of the nervous system. Neuron 1988;**1**:623–634

[50] Head BP, Patel HH, Niesman IR, Drummond JC, Roth DM, Patel PM: Inhibition of p75 neurotrophin receptor attenuates isoflurane-mediated neuronal apoptosis in the neonatal central nervous system. Anesthesiology 2009;**110**:813–825

[51] Elmore S: Apoptosis: a review of programmed cell death. Toxicol Pathol 2007;**35**: 495–516

[52] Hays SR, Deshpande JK: Newly postulated neurodevelopmental risks of pediatric anesthesia: theories that could rock our world. J Urol 2013;**189**:1222–1228

[53] Reddy SV: Effect of general anesthetics on the developing brain. J Anaesthesiol Clin Pharmacol. 2012;**28**:6–10.

[54] Twaroski D, Bosnjak ZJ, Bai X. MicroRNAs: new players in anesthetic-induced developmental neurotoxicity. Pharm Anal Acta. 2015;**6**:357.

[55] Twaroski DM, Yan Y, Olson JM, Bosnjak ZJ, Bai X: Down-regulation of microRNA-21 is involved in the propofol-induced neurotoxicity observed in human stem cell-derived neurons. Anesthesiology 2014;**121**:786–800.

[56] Huang C, Zhang X, Zheng J, Chen C, Chen Y, Yi J: Upregulation of miR-137 protects anesthesia-induced hippocampal neurodegeneration. Int J Clin Exp Pathol 2014;**7**:5000–5007.

[57] Mintz CD, Wagner M, Loepke AW: Preclinical research into the effects of anesthetics on the developing brain: promises and pitfalls. J Neurosurg Anesthesiol. 2012;**24**:362–367.

[58] Luo L: Actin cytoskeleton regulation in neuronal morphogenesis and structural plasticity. Annu Rev Cell Dev Biol. 2002;**18**:601–635

[59] Jevtovic-Todorovic V: Anesthesia and the developing brain: are we getting closer to understanding the truth? Curr Opin Anaesthesiol. 2011;**24**:395–399

[60] Jin H, Hu Z, Dong M, Wu Y, Zhu Z, Xu L: Ketamine induces tau hyperphosphorylation at serine 404 in the hippocampus of neonatal rats. Neural Regen Res. 2013;**8**:1590–1596.

[61] Guilarte TR, Chen MK: Translocator protein 18 kDa (TSPO): molecular sensor of brain injury and repair. Pharmacol Ther 2008;**118**:1–17.

[62] Perera F, Herbstman J: Prenatal environmental exposures, epigenetics and disease. Reprod Toxicol. 2011;**31**:363–373.

[63] Olsen EA, Brambrink AM: Anesthesia for the young child undergoing ambulatory procedures: current concerns regarding harm to the developing brain. Curr Opin Anesthesiol 2013;**26**:677–684

[64] Pellegrini L, Bennis Y, Velly L, Grandvuillemin I, Pisano P, Bruder N, et al: Erythropoietin protects newborn rat against sevoflurane-induced neurotoxicity. Paediatr Anaesth. 2014;**24**:749–759.

[65] Vutskits L, Davis PJ, Hansen TG: Anesthetics and the developing brain: time for a change in practice? A pro/con debate. Pediatr Anesth 2012;**22**:973–980

[66] Sander RD, Davidson A: Anesthetic-induced neurotoxicity of the neonate: time for clinical guidelines? Pediatr Anesth 2009;**19**:1141–1146

[67] Flick RP, Katusic SK, Colligan RC, Wilder RT, Voigt RG, Olson MD, et al: Cognitive and behavioral outcomes after early exposure to anesthesia and surgery. Pediatrics. 2011;**128**:e1053–e1061.

[68] Sprung J, Flick RP, Katusic SK, Colligan RC, Barbaresi WJ, Bojanić K, et al: Attention-deficit/hyperactivity disorder after early exposure to procedures requiring general anesthesia. Mayo Clin Proc. 2012;**87**:120–129.

[69] Flick RP, Lee K, Hofer RE, Beinborn CW, Hambel EM, Klein MK, et al: Neuraxial labor analgesia for vaginal delivery and its effects on childhood learning disabilities. Anesth Analg. 2011;**112**:1424–1431

[70] Sprung J, Flick RP, Wilder RT, Katusic SK, Pike TL, Dingli M, et al: Anesthesia for cesarean delivery and learning disabilities in a population-based birth cohort. Anesthesiology. 2009;**111**:302–310.

[71] DiMaggio C, Sun LS, Li G: Early childhood exposure to anesthesia and risk of developmental and behavioral disorders in a sibling birth cohort. Anesth Analg. 2011;**113**:1143–1151

[72] Meyer P, Langlois C, Soëte S, Leydet J, Echenne B, Rivier F, et al: Unexpected neurological sequelae following propofol anesthesia in infants: three case reports. Brain Dev 2010;**32**:872–878

[73] Fresofol product information. Available from: http://www.fresenius-kabi.com.au/files/Fresofol_PI.pdf

http://dx.doi.org/10.5772/65921

[74] Gleich SJ, Flick R, Hu D, Zaccariello MJ, Colligan RC, Katusic SK, et al: Neurodevelopment of children exposed to anesthesia: design of the mayo anesthesia safety in kids (MASK) study. Contemp Clin Trials 2015;**41**:45–54

[75] Sun LS, Li G, DiMaggio CJ, Byrne MW, Ing C, Miller TL, et al: Feasibility and pilot study of the pediatric anesthesia neurodevelopment assessment (PANDA) project. J Neurosurg Anesthesiol. 2012;**24**:382–388.

[76] Miller TL, Park R, Sun LS: Report of the third PANDA symposium on "Anesthesia and Neurodevelopment in Children". J Neurosurg Anesthesiol. 2012;**24**:357–361

[77] Byrne MW, Ascherman JA, Casale P, Cowles RA, Gallin PF, Maxwell LG: Elective procedures and anesthesia in children: pediatric surgeons enter the dialogue on neurotoxicity questions, surgical options, and parental concerns. J Neurosurg Anesthesiol. 2012;**24**:396–400.

[78] Miller TL, Park R, Sun LS: Report of the fourth PANDA symposium on "anesthesia and neurodevelopment in children". J Neurosurg Anesthesiol. 2014;**26**:344–348.

[79] Jevtovic-Todorovic V: Pediatric anesthesia neurotoxicity: an overview of the 2011 SmartTots panel. Anesth Analg 2011;**113**:965–968

[80] Davidson AJ, Disma N, de Graaff JC, Withington DE, Dorris L, Bell G, et al: Neurodevelopmental outcome at 2 years of age after general anaesthesia and awake-regional anaesthesia in infancy (GAS): an international multicentre, randomised controlled trial. Lancet. 2016;**387**:239–250

[81] Nemergut ME, Aganga D, Flick RP: Anesthetic neurotoxicity: what to tell the parents? Pediatr Anesth 2014;**24**:120–126

Preoperative Evaluation of Computed Tomography Perfusion: Its Significance for the Risk Assessment of Cerebrovascular Complications Perioperatively[1]

Yusuke Asakura, Yuta Matsunaga, Maho Kinoshita, Yusuke Kasuya and Makoto Ozaki

Additional information is available at the end of the chapter

http://dx.doi.org/10.5772/65724

Abstract

Neurological complications occur with an overall frequency of 2.8% perioperatively. Although ultrasound imaging is an excellent modality for the risk assessment of carotid arterial diseases, no comprehensive information can be obtained with respect to the intracranial cerebral blood flow. Recent advent of computed tomography perfusion (CTP) imaging has made it possible to directly measure the cerebral blood flow at any intracranial region of interest. We describe here an efficacy of CT perfusion imaging in the preoperative settings for the risk assessment of neurological complications, especially in cases with carotid arterial stenosis/occlusion.

Keywords: computed tomography perfusion, cerebral blood flow, carotid arterial stenosis

1. Introduction

Although overall mortality for patients undergoing coronary bypass graft surgery (CABG) has decreased by 23% in 1990s, the incidence of stroke perioperatively has remained unchanged [1]. Some report suggests that perioperative neurological complications occur with

[1] This work was in part presented at the 33rd Annual Congress of the Scandinavian Society of Anesthesiology and Intensive Care Medicine, Reykjavik, Iceland, 2015, and the 62nd Annual Congress of Japanese Society of Anesthesiologists, 2015, Kobe, Japan.

an overall frequency of 2.8%, and an incidence rate of 0.9% in patients younger than 65 years, 3.6% aged between 65 and 74 years, and 8.9% older than 75 years [2]. Additionally, the patient with a neurological complication has a ninefold increase in mortality [2]. Carotid arterial disease accounts for approximately 10% of perioperative cerebral complications [3]. Although ultrasound imaging is an excellent modality for evaluating the morphology of the carotid arteries with its excellent spatial resolution [3], intracranial cerebral blood flow dynamics cannot be assessed by the use of ultrasound. Here, we report that computed tomography perfusion (CTP) imaging is an efficacious modality for evaluating the intracranial cerebral flow.

In our facility, CTP imaging has been introduced in 2012, and 58 cases underwent its evaluation by the end of 2014. After obtaining an IRB (Institutional Review Board) approval, we have analyzed all the 58 cases, and identified 11 individuals who have been diagnosed as having carotid arterial stenosis/occlusion. We have measured cerebral blood flow (CBF), cerebral blood volume (CBV), and mean transit time (MTT) at the ipsilateral as well as at the contralateral hemisphere, and their correlation to the subsequent development of neurological events during the 2-year follow-up period was evaluated.

Of 11 patients, the decreased CBF at the ipsilateral hemisphere was noted in four individuals, and the other seven showed intact CTP findings. All the four patients who showed decreased CBF pattern and the one who showed normal CTP finding developed cerebrovascular diseases during the 2-year follow-up period. The rest of six individuals who showed normal CTP findings have remained otherwise healthy. We suggest that the decreased CBF at the ipsilateral side may predict the possible neurological complications in the patients with carotid arterial stenosis/occlusion. In patients with carotid arterial stenosis whose cerebral blood flow (CBF) has remained intact, the patients' outcome has remained favorable, and they have remained otherwise healthy. By contrast, in patients whose CBF is decreased, they have developed severe cerebrovascular complications. The findings described here potentially indicate the possibility that CT perfusion findings may predict the perioperative outcomes in patients with carotid arterial stenosis/occlusion.

2. Computed tomography perfusion

CT perfusion is a new technique which enables to evaluate both rapid qualitative and quantitative cerebral perfusion by means of generating cerebral blood flow (CBF), cerebral blood volume (CBV), and mean transit time (MTT) [4]. Thus far, several modalities such as magnetic resonance (MR) perfusion [5], xenon computed tomography (xenon CT) [6], positron emission tomography (PET) [7], and single photon emission computed tomography (SPECT) [8] have been used to evaluate cerebral perfusion. Compared to these modalities, CT perfusion can be performed easily and quickly by the use of any standard spiral CT scanner in patients where unenhanced CT is planned to exclude acute intracranial hemorrhage. The fundamental theory of this technique is the central volume principle [4]. It correlates cerebral blood flow (CBF) with cerebral blood volume (CBV) and mean transit time (MTT) in the following equation: CBF =

CBV/MTT. In brief, by monitoring the first pass of an iodinated contrast agent by the bolus injection through the cerebral vasculature, the linear relationship between contrast agent concentration and attenuation can be obtained in a given region of interest. After an acquisition of the raw results, data are analyzed at an imaging workstation (Advantage Windows; GE Medical Systems) equipped with commercially available software (CT perfusion; GE Medical Systems). By the use of CT perfusion, it becomes easy and quick to identify and quantify the presence and extent of a perfusion deficit in an acute stroke setting in whom an emergent thrombolytic therapy is going to be considered [9]. In addition, it is also suitable for the evaluation of cerebrovascular reserve in patients with stenotic lesions who would be the potential candidates for neuroendovascular treatment and bypass surgery.

Although other multi-modalities such as SPECT/CT and PET/CT system also provide good comprehensive information with respect to the combination of anatomical and functional data, they usually require the specific equipment which sometimes makes it difficult to their global diffusion into the clinical practice [7, 8]. For instance, for SPECT/CT, a dual-detector gamma camera and a low-dose four-slice CT mounted on the same rotate platform are required (Infinia Hawkeye 4, GE Medical Systems). By contrast, CT perfusion can be performed easily and quickly using a standard spiral CT scanner and does not require specific equipment except for an imaging workstation, which makes it suitable for the global use in the evaluation of cerebral blood flow.

3. CT perfusion may predict patients' outcome in patients with carotid arterial stenosis

Except for a history of hypertension, an otherwise healthy 72-year-old male was planned for an elective surgery for his cervical disc hernia. His preoperative evaluation of carotid ultrasonography revealed total occlusion of the left internal carotid artery (**Figure 1A**). Since we have experienced a similar case in which stroke has developed shortly after the diagnosis of total occlusion of the left internal carotid artery (**Figure 1B**), we planned to evaluate the potential risks of developing neurological complications perioperatively by CT perfusion. In the latter case in which stroke has been confirmed soon after the diagnosis of total left internal carotid artery occlusion, simultaneous evaluation of CT perfusion revealed clear laterality of cerebral blood flow imaging, suggesting that the left intracranial hypoperfusion was apparent owing to the total occlusion of the left internal carotid artery (**Figure 1C**). By contrast, in the former case, no laterality of the intracranial cerebral flow was observed, suggesting that the collateral circulation may have compensated the total occlusion of the left internal carotid artery (**Figure 1D**). To further confirm that there is no laterality of cerebral blood flow between the right and the left hemispheres, we calculated the cerebral blood flow (CBF), mean transit time (MTT), and the cerebral blood volume (CBV) in his both hemispheres. The right cerebral blood flow was 34.4 mL/100 g/min and the left CBF was 34.5 mL/100 g/min. The cerebral blood volume (CBV) of his right hemisphere was 2.7 mL/100 g and the CBV of his left hemisphere was 2.9 mL/100 g. The mean transit time (MTT) of his right hemisphere was 4.9 s and the left was 5.3

s. The results clearly showed that there was no difference between his right and left hemispheres with respect to the dynamics of cerebral blood flow, although prolonged MTT was equally observed in both hemispheres to some degree. Based on the results of CT perfusion, the patient was given the consent that if his neurological symptoms relating to his cervical disc hernia would further worsen, he is going to be scheduled for an elective surgery. During the 2-year follow-up period, he has not developed any cerebrovascular complications and has remained otherwise healthy.

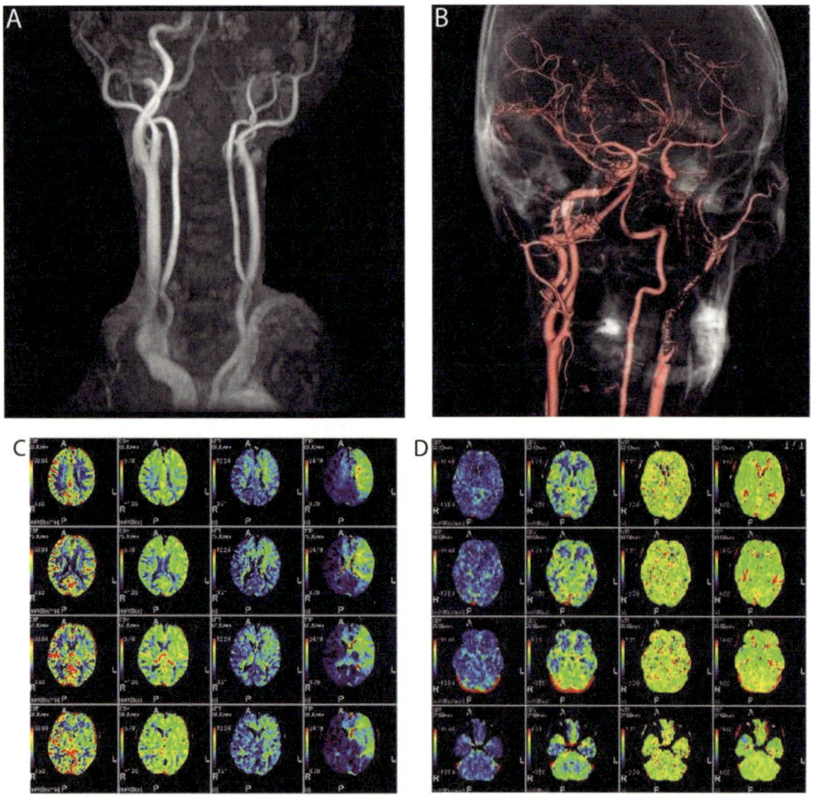

Figure 1. (**A**) A 72-year-old male presented to our hospital complaining the pain in the left upper extremity. He was diagnosed as having cervical disc hernia. Simultaneous evaluation of cervical MR angiography together with ultrasound imaging revealed total occlusion of the left internal carotid artery. (**B**) A 65-year-old male presented to our hospital because of transient gait instability and dysarthria. CT angiography together with ultrasound imaging revealed total occlusion of the left internal carotid artery. (**C**) CT perfusion imaging revealed an apparent decrease of CBF and prolonged MTT in his left hemisphere. (**D**) CT perfusion imaging of the 72-year-old male revealed no apparent laterality of CBF, CBV, and MTT between the right and the left hemispheres.

After obtaining Institutional Review Board's approval, we have further surveyed all the medical charts of 58 patients who have been examined by CT perfusion in our facility between 2012 and 2014. Among the 58 cases, we have identified 11 individuals who have been diagnosed as having carotid arterial stenosis by ultrasonography. Among 11 patients with carotid arterial stenosis, 7 patients had no apparent CBF laterality or CBV laterality. Except for one case in whom bilateral carotid arterial stenosis (77% stenosis in the right internal carotid artery and 85% stenosis in the left carotid artery) was noted by ultrasonography who subsequently was found dead at his home, all the six cases have remained otherwise healthy without any cerebrovascular complications during the 2-year follow-up period, which suggests that the intact CT perfusion findings may predict favorable outcome in patients with carotid arterial stenosis (**Table 1**). By contrast, the rest of four patients with an apparent CBF decrease either with maintained CBV or with decreased CBV developed irreversible cerebrovascular complications either at the time of evaluation of CT perfusion or during the 2-year follow-up period (**Table 1**). The incidence of development of cerebrovascular complication was significantly higher in whom an abnormal CT perfusion finding was observed ($p = 0.006$, chi-squared test).

	Decreased CBF at the ipsilateral hemisphere	Intact CT perfusion findings
The number of patients who developed irreversible cerebrovascular complications	4	1*
The number of patients who remained otherwise healthy without neurological symptoms	0	6**

Among 11 patients who were diagnosed as having carotid arterial stenosis by ultrasonography, 4 patients showed an apparent decreased CBF at the ipsilateral hemisphere, and 7 patients showed normal CT perfusion findings. All the four patients developed irreversible cerebrovascular complications either at the time when CT perfusion was evaluated or during the 2-year follow-up period.
*Bilateral carotid arterial stenosis (77% stenosis in the right internal carotid artery and 85% stenosis in the left carotid artery) was noted by ultrasonography, and the patient was subsequently found dead at his home.
**Although the sample power is not strong enough, the likelihood of the patients with carotid arterial stenosis to remain healthy appeared to have correlated with their intact CT perfusion findings ($p = 0.006$, chi-squared test).

Table 1. The outcome of the patients with carotid arterial stenosis (with 2-year follow-up) and its correlation to their findings of CT perfusion.

4. Delayed hypocerebral perfusion following aneurysmal clipping surgery: A new clinical entity

Among 58 cases, we found five individuals who had undergone neurosurgical clipping for subarachnoid hemorrhage either at our facility or in the other hospital. Notably, two out of five cases were found to have hypoperfusion of cerebral blood flow at the distal regions of artery where clipping was performed. A 72-year-old female underwent neurosurgical clipping of the right mid-cerebral artery due to the ruptured aneurysm at the age of 58 at the other hospital (**Figure 2A**). Eleven years after surgery, she presented at our hospital, complaining of right tinnitus, vertigo, and headache. She was eventually evaluated by CT angiography together with CT perfusion, which revealed an apparent hypoperfusion of the right mid-cerebral artery (**Figure 2B**). Her cerebral blood flow corresponding to the region where the right mid-cerebral artery perfuses is 16.4 mL/100 g/min, whereas the cerebral blood flow of the contralateral hemisphere was 32.7 mL/100 g/min. The CBV corresponding to the right mid-cerebral artery is 1.0 mL/100 g and the CBV of the contralateral hemisphere was 1.1 mL/100 g.

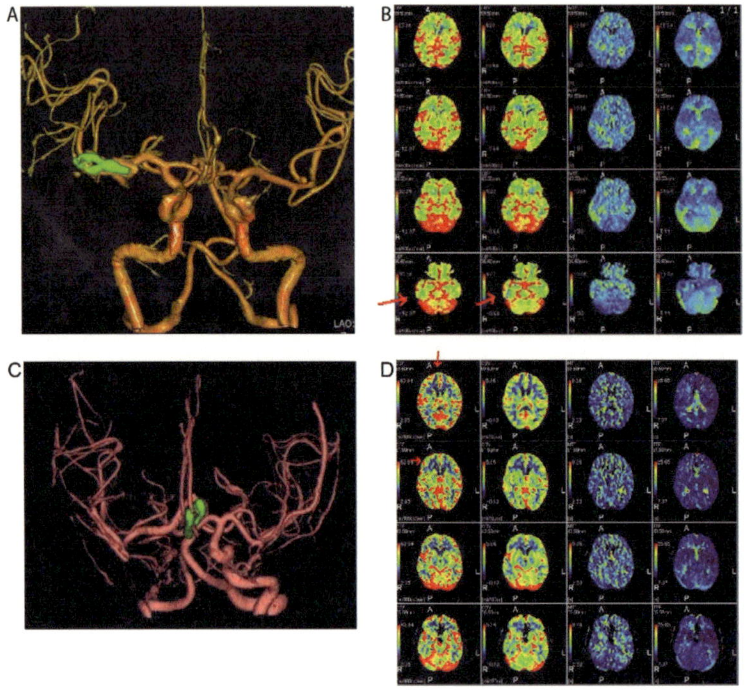

Figure 2. (**A**) A 72-year-old female underwent neurosurgical clipping of the right mid-cerebral artery due to the ruptured aneurysm at the age of 58 at the other hospital. Her CT angiography is shown in the figure. (**B**) CT perfusion findings revealed an apparent decrease of cerebral blood flow perfused by the right mid-cerebral artery (indicated by the arrows). (**C**) A 63-year-old woman underwent emergent neuroclipping surgery for the ruptured anterior-communicating artery aneurysm. Her CT angiography is shown in the figure. The surgery is successfully carried out. (**D**) Six months postoperatively, a physiotherapist noticed her slight memory defect, and CT perfusion was evaluated, which revealed an apparent hypoperfusion of both frontal lobes (indicated by the arrows).

The right MTT was 4.6 s and the left MTT was 4.6 s, confirming the results that the cerebral blood flow of the right mid-cerebral artery just distal of the clipped region is actually decreasing. Similarly, a 63-year-old woman underwent emergent clipping surgery for the ruptured anterior-communicating artery aneurysm (**Figure 2C**). During the follow-up period, she had a slight defect of memory, and the CT perfusion was evaluated, which clearly revealed the impairment of cerebral blood flow in both the frontal lobes (**Figure 2D**). The quantification of the cerebral blood flow actually confirmed the decrease of the cerebral blood flow in both the frontal lobes as compared to the regions where mid-cerebral artery perfuses (CBF; right frontal: 17.1 mL/100 g/min, left frontal: 14.1 mL/100 g/min; right temporal: 43.5 mL/100 g/min, left temporal: 48.4 mL/100 g/min). The significance of the findings is that although anesthesiologists usually consider the patients who had successfully undergone neuroclipping surgery as the standard risk group, we found here that they still may pose a risk for neurological complications perioperatively even after the successful surgery. The finding may encompasses not only to the perioperative risks of patients who had undergone aneurysmal clipping surgery but also to its delayed neurological manifestations associated with the hypoperfusion of parental artery, a possible new diagnostic clinical entity.

5. Computed tomography perfusion as the means to noninvasively measure tumor malignancy

Tumors usually exhibit increased angiogenic activity and neovascularization, which result in increased blood volume. Accordingly, previous studies suggested that CBV and CBF were elevated in tumors, and they may be efficacious in the assessment of tumor angiogenic activity.

A 59-year-old male visited our hospital complaining of dizziness and nausea. His T2-weighed magnetic resonance image showed an overt edematous left temporal lobe (**Figure 3A**). Based on the images obtained, the presence of limbic encephalitis was suspected. He was coincidentally seropositive for human T-cell leukemia virus-1 (HTLV-1). Accordingly, the other differential diagnosis such as non-Hodgkin lymphoma, limbic encephalitis associated with autoimmunity, paraneoplastic syndrome (PNLE; paraneoplastic limbic encephalitis), herpes encephalitis, and astrocytoma could also be possible. In an attempt to obtain further clues for the diagnosis of his disease, especially to determine whether or not directly to obtain histopathological findings by craniotomy, CT perfusion study was performed. The CT perfusion findings indicated a moderate increase of CBV in the corresponding region (**Figure 3B**), an apparent increase of TTP (time to peak) (**Figure 3B**), a slight increase of MTT, and an intact CBF (**Figure 3B**), which indicates the potential possibility of the presence of the primary tumor surrounded by the edematous normal brain tissue. Based on the findings, he underwent computer-navigated craniotomy. The postoperative histopathological findings confirmed the presence of astrocytoma grade 2.

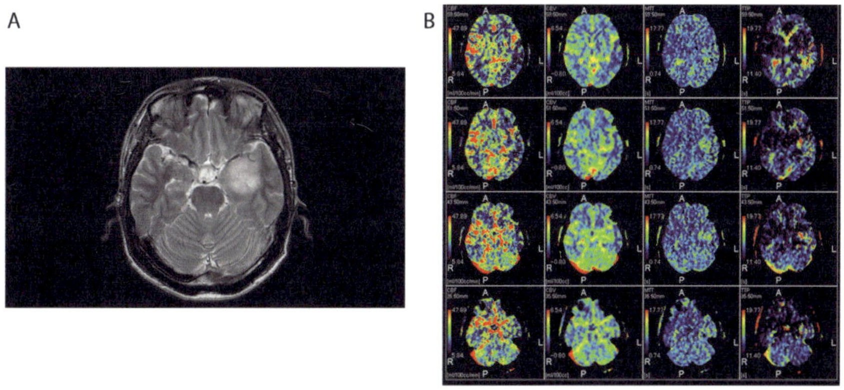

Figure 3. (**A**) T2-weighed magnetic resonance image of a 59-year-old male who presented to our hospital because of dizziness and nausea. An edematous region of the temporal lobe is apparent, suggesting the presence of limbic encephalitis. (**B**) A CT perfusion imaging of the same patient. From left to the right, CBF, CBV, MTT, and TTP are visualized. The corresponding region where limbic encephalitis is suspected, an apparent increase of CBV and TTP is observed. CBF remained intact and a slight increase of MTT is also observed.

Since an increase of CBV and TTP reflects angiogenic activity and neovascularization of the tumor, our findings may indicate that CT perfusion findings may potentially be predictive of pathologic grade of the tumor and correlate with tumor mitotic activity. Because the diagnosis of limbic encephalitis is extremely difficult and the laboratory investigations often only provide inconclusive evidence, we suggest that CT perfusion is potentially an important modality that may provide clues to the correct diagnosis.

6. Implications of the study results

We have shown here that the CT perfusion is an efficacious modality to evaluate the intracranial cerebral blood flow dynamics and may predict the favorable outcome in the cases with carotid arterial stenosis whose CT perfusion findings have remained intact. Using the standard 16-section multidetector scanners, CT perfusion together with CT angiography can be rapidly performed in less than 2 min. CT perfusion can measure virtually every brain tissue blood perfusion, and the commonly used parameters in CT perfusion are as follows: CBF: cerebral blood flow, CBV: cerebral blood volume, and MTT: mean transit time. CBF is defined as the flowing blood volume moving through a given volume (usually 100 g) of brain in a specific amount of time. CBV is defined as the flowing blood volume in the given volume of brain. MTT is defined as the average amount of time the blood takes to transit through the given volume of brain.

CT perfusion has come to its clinical use in the mid-2000s and it has now a growing role in the evaluation of intracranial hemodynamics [9–11]. The tissue that shows decreased CBF with maintained CBV indicates those with severe hypoperfusion. The tissue that shows decreased CBF with decreased CBV and increased MTT suggests those with irreversible ischemic change. Although the number of patients we were able to evaluate was limited, it appears likely that those with intact CT perfusion findings have apparent good prognosis irrespective of the presence of carotid stenosis.

In conclusion, by using CT perfusion, it appears feasible to evaluate the intracranial cerebral flow dynamics which is difficult to assess by the use of ultrasound, and it may predict the favorable outcome if the CT perfusion findings have remained intact. The findings described here would further contribute to the preoperative evaluation of the risk assessment of potential devastating neurological complications, especially for those undergoing cardiac surgeries. We also suggest that in patients with carotid arterial stenosis, the evaluation of CT perfusion in the preoperative settings would be the prerequisite for the avoidance of possible development of cerebrovascular complications perioperatively.

Acknowledgements

We thank Mr. Hiroaki Okuzawa, Dr. Hisato Nakazawa, and Ms. Sawayo Kinoshita, Department of Radiology, Nagoya Kyoritsu Hospital, for their excellent technical assistance. Support was provided solely by institutional sources.

http://dx.doi.org/10.5772/65724

Author details

Yusuke Asakura[1*], Yuta Matsunaga[2], Maho Kinoshita[3], Yusuke Kasuya[3] and Makoto Ozaki[3]

*Address all correspondence to: yasakura@kaikou.or.jp

1 Department of Anesthesiology, Nagoya Kyoritsu Hospital, Nagoya, Japan

2 Department of Radiology, Nagoya Kyoritsu Hospital, Nagoya, Japan

3 Tokyo Women's Medical University, Tokyo, Japan

References

[1] Fergusson TB Jr, Hammill BG, Peterson ED, DeLong ER Grover FL; STS National Database Committee. A decade of change-risk profiles and outcomes for isolated coronary artery bypass grafting procedures, 1990–1999: A report from the STS National Database Committee and the Duke Clinical Research Institute. Society of Thoracic Surgeons. Ann Thorac Surg 2002; 73: 480–9.

[2] Tunman KJ, McCarthy RJ, Najafi H, et al. Differential effects of advanced age on neurologic and cardiac risks of coronary artery operations. J Thorac Cardiovasc Surg 1992; 104; 1510.

[3] Asakura Y, Nakamichi Y, Mori K, Ibuki K, Kasuga H, Hori H. Ultrasound-guided central venous catheterization: efficacy of simultaneous perioperative ultrasonographic scanning for the presence of carotid plaques in the prevention of the perioperative development of ischemic stroke. J Anesth 2012; 26; 621–2.

[4] Koenig M, Klotz E, Luka B, Venderink DJ, Spittler JF, Heuser L. Perfusion CT of the brain: diagnostic approach for early detection of ischemic stroke. Radiology 1998; 209: 85–93.

[5] Provenzale JM, Shah K, Patel U, McCrony DC. Systematic review of CT and MR perfusion imaging for assessment of acute cerebrovascular disease. AJNR Am J Neuroradiol 2008; 29: 1476–82.

[6] Johnston DW, Stringer WA, Marks MP, Yonas H, Good WF, Gur D. Stable xenon CT cerebral blood flow imaging: rationale for and role in clinical decision making. AJNR Am J Neuroradiol 1991 12: 201–13.

[7] Cavalcanti Fiho JL, de Souza Leao Lima R, de Souza Machado Neo L, Kayatto Bittencourt L, Domingues RC, da Fanseca ML. PET/CT and vascular disease: current concepts. Eur J Radiol 2011; 80: 60–7.

[8] Mariani G, Brusseli L, Kuwert T, Kim EE, Flotats A, Israel O, Dondi M, Watanabe N. A review on the clinical uses of SPECT/CT. Eur J Nucl Med Mol Imaging 2010; 37: 1959–85.

[9] Hoeffner EG, Case I, Jain R, Gujar SK, Shah GV, Deveikis JP, Carlos RC, Thompson BG, Harrigan MR, Mukherji SK. Cerebral perfusion CT: technique and clinical applications. Radiology 2004; 231: 632–44.

[10] Lui YW, Tang ER, Allmendinger AM, Spektor V. Evaluation of CT perfusion in the settings of cerebral ischemia: patterns and pitfalls. Am J Neuroradiol 2010; 31: 1552–63.

[11] Mair G, Wardlaw JM. Imaging of acute stroke prior to treatment: current practice and evolving techniques. Br J Radiol 2014; 87: 20140216.

Chapter 7

Postoperative Cognitive Dysfunction: Preclinical Highlights and Perspectives on Preventive Strategies

Fabricio M. Locatelli and Takashi Kawano

Additional information is available at the end of the chapter

http://dx.doi.org/10.5772/66574

Abstract

One of the common complications associated with anaesthesia and surgery in geriatric patients is the postoperative cognitive dysfunction (POCD). This cognitive impairment affects the long-term prognosis and has been shown to be associated with long-term disability, higher health care costs, and even increased mortality. On the other hand, clinical research on POCD is in its infancy, the condition has not been clarified, and since no strategy for management is currently available, it is imperative to develop specific methods for prevention and management. Although its pathogenesis involves various factors, accumulating evidence suggests that surgery elicits an inflammatory response in the hippocampus, a brain area closely related to cognitive function, playing a key role in the development of POCD. Several studies suggest that age-related phenotypic change of microglia is associated with pathogenic neuroinflammation, and more importantly it may be modifiable. In this chapter, we discuss the current overview and preclinical highlights regarding POCD. We further discuss some perspectives on preventive strategies for POCD, based on the findings of our preclinical research and the available literature.

Keywords: POCD, neuroinflammation, microglia

1. Introduction

Sixty years ago, an article entitled *Adverse cerebral effects of anaesthesia on old people* by Dr. Bedfor was published in which he reported for the first time that general anaesthesia and surgery led to cognitive dysfunction in elderly patients [1]. This decline, known as postoperative cognitive dysfunction (POCD), typically persists for several weeks, sometimes a year, but in some people is permanent. Since then, the number of publications assessing POCD has been growing year by year, reflecting the increasing importance and the still remaining controversies over this condition [2].

One of the greatest achievements of modern medicine is the increase in life expectancy; however, as a consequence the world population is today ageing fast, with over 12.3% of the total being over 60 years old [3]. Moreover, life expectancy increased by 5 years between 2000 and 2015, the fastest growth since the 1960s [4]. Though it is one of our greatest achievements, it also poses big challenges as the ageing process is associated with biological and cognitive degeneration [5]. Recent advances in surgical, anaesthetic management and intensive care techniques are associated with a growing number of elderly people undergoing surgical procedures [6]. Consequently, complications associated with geriatric surgery, such as POCD, will become an increasingly common worldwide problem [7, 8]. Furthermore, POCD has been shown to be associated with long-term disability and higher health care costs. In addition, three-month POCD has been statistically associated with increased mortality [9].

POCD is difficult to define; in general it refers to a deterioration in cognition that occurs in the time period after surgery. To truly diagnose POCD, it is necessary to have tested the patient preoperatively (baseline) and determined how much of a decline occurred after surgery. As can be expected, in normal clinical contexts, patients do not usually undergo neuropsychological testing pre- and post-surgery [2, 10]. In consequence, there is a lack of accurate data and even the exact incidence of this condition is unknown [10]. Besides, behavioral responses to cognitive tests not only vary considerably in aged individuals compared with younger individuals, but also an enormous variability of cognitive decline exists across individuals [6, 11]. Additionally, the changes produced by the effects of ageing on cognitive function vary substantially through the different cognitive domains [11]. Likewise, different cognitive domains must be evaluated by specific tests [2]. Hence in order to diagnose and characterize POCD cases, it becomes necessary to carry out neuropsychological tests that assess different domains involved in cognitive function such as learning and memory, attention, psychomotor function and flexibility cognition [2, 10]. In addition, POCD is sometimes characterized by slight declines in cognitive function, making it essential that these tests should be sensitive enough to allow an accurate diagnosis based on the results of pre-and postoperative tests [10]. As a consequence, incidence rates reported may vary considerably according to the cognitive domains explored by different tests and timing [12].

POCD was initially associated with cardiac surgery and indeed was recognized as the most common complication in this intervention, presenting a high incidence [13, 14], although the incidence values vary considerably between different reports, ranging from approximately 30% to 80% at the time of discharge, 10–60% after 3–6 months and 20–60% after 6 months to 1 year [12–20]. This fact may be related to microembolic events that may cause focal cerebral infarcts during the use of the cardiopulmonary bypass pump [12, 21–24].

In recent times, in correlation with the continuingly increasing number of patients undergoing geriatric surgery, the interest in POCD has expanded to noncardiac surgery as well. So far, the major study assessing this condition was carried out by the International Study of Postoperative Cognitive Dysfunction and included 1218 patients older than 60 years old undergoing elective, noncardiac surgery [7]. Neuropsychological tests were administered before surgery and at 7 days and 3 months after intervention. This study reported a POCD incidence of 25% 1 week after surgery and 10% after 3 months. Additionally, the probability of POCD incidence in patients aged 70 and over at 3 months (14%) was two times higher than those aged 60 to 69 (7%). Hovens and collaborators [25] reported that the cognitive domains affected by cardiac surgery compared with noncardiac surgery seem to be different. While abdominal surgery affects hippocampal neuronal functioning and in consequence spatial memory, cardiac surgery seems to cause a more general change in inflammation and neuronal function [25].

Furthermore, there appears to exist an association between postoperative pain and cognitive impairment, exerting an influence over the patients' performance on certain cognitive tests [26–28]. Apart from the effect of the pain, the influence of postoperative analgesics should not be ruled out. In fact, successful postoperative pain management may be important in preventing POCD in elderly patients [35]. Additionally, cognitive impairment in elderly patients may also be influenced by stress produced by the hospitalization itself, the postoperative fatigue state, the unfamiliar environment and sleep deprivation [12, 28, 29].

The contribution of the anaesthesia to the development of POCD seems to be subject to discrepancies. When Silbert and colleagues [30] assessed general anaesthesia compared with spinal anaesthesia, no significant difference in the rates of POCD was found. In agreement with this, a meta-analysis carried on by Guay [31] did not find differences between general anaesthesia and regional anaesthesia with spontaneous breathing and sedation only in the development of permanent POCD after noncardiac surgery. Otherwise, another meta-analysis concluded that general anaesthesia, compared to other types of anaesthesia, may increase the risk of developing POCD [32]. This findings are supported by preclinical studies, which suggest that isoflurane anaesthesia administered at clinically relevant doses causes long-term cognitive impairment in unoperated animals [33–35]. However, other studies point towards an enhancement of the cognitive functions after anaesthesia inhalation [36–38].

Although major surgery is frequently associated with the development of POCD, minor surgery proved to decrease the cognitive function in the first postoperative week in elderly patients [39]. Moreover, independently from the nature of the surgical procedure, the only consistent risk factor that has been identified for POCD is advanced age [7, 9, 15, 39–41]. Apart from increasing age as a risk factor for POCD, other factors that can be enumerated are lower level of education, a history of previous cerebral vascular accident, a history of alcohol dependence, preoperative history of post-traumatic stress disorder, poor cognitive health, preceding development of POCD, respiratory complications, infectious complications and a second operation [9, 12, 41–43].

2. Mechanisms of POCD

One of the most challenging problems connected with POCD is the lack of evidence-based preventative strategies. This is due to the fact that the mechanisms that cause POCD in elderly patients are largely unknown. In fact, surgery induces peripheral immune challenges, leading to an exaggerated neuroinflammatory response. More recently, several studies have demonstrated that neuroinflammation in the hippocampus is most likely to be involved in the pathogenesis of POCD [35, 44–51]. Neuroinflammation is a complex response to brain injury characterized by maladaptive microglial activation mainly involving the activation of glia and increased levels of pro-inflammatory cytokines, including interleukin-1β (IL-1β) and tumour necrosis factor-α (TNF-α) [52–54]. As the primary source for pro-inflammatory cytokines, microglia are implicated as pivotal mediators of neuroinflammation. In particular, the hippocampus is known to be a region important to cognition and highly vulnerable to ageing. Pro-inflammatory cytokines TNF-α and IL-1β released from microglia within the hippocampus are reported to inhibit the long-term potentiation that is important in the formation of memory, as well as inducing apoptosis, and thus play a pathogenic role in cognitive disorders in neurodegenerative diseases [48, 52–58]. Based on these findings, it can be hypothesized that age-related microglial priming in the hippocampus, and subsequent overproduction of inflammatory cytokines, plays a critical role in the development of POCD in the elderly population. Therefore, it becomes necessary to understand the roles of neuroinflammation in the pathogenesis of POCD and its potential as a therapeutic target.

Preclinical evidence has shown that microglia in a normal-aged brain are shifted towards the inflammatory phenotype (**Figure 1**). This age-related phenotype change is consistent with the microglial priming, implying that age-related microglia priming could make elderly surgical patients more susceptible to the development of POCD. Neurogenic neuroinflammation is the inflammatory reaction in the central nervous system in response to neuronal activity [59]. Peripheral immune challenges, such as surgical trauma, may lead neurogenic neuroinflammation to become maladaptive [60]. It has been postulated that the inflammatory response may be transmitted through humoral and neural pathways, leading to neuroinflammation. Parabiotic experiments in rat models have revealed that the neural pathway may play a dominant role in the development of neuroinflammation after abdominal surgery [60]. These findings seem to confirm the neurogenic neuroinflammatory origin of POCD in aged rats. Though rodents are useful in providing hypothetical models for understanding some of the memory deficits seen in human POCD, it still remains unclear how much can be extrapolated to simulate the neuroinflammatory mechanisms involved in human POCD [2].

While several studies have concentrated on protein regulating inflammation (cytokines), recent evidence points to a critical role of microRNAs (miRNAs) in controlling the inflammatory process [61–64]. A subset of miRNAs notably affects both immune and neuronal functions in particular in the central nervous system. It has been hypothesized that miRNAs regulate neuro-immune functions through alterations of neuron-glia and/or brain-to-body signalling [65]. Moreover, miR-572 has been implicated in the development and restoration of POCD and identified as a possible biological marker for early diagnosis of POCD [61]. In fact, modulating miRNAs using agonist or antagonist miRNAs is a promising approach to treating human neuroinflammatory disorders including POCD.

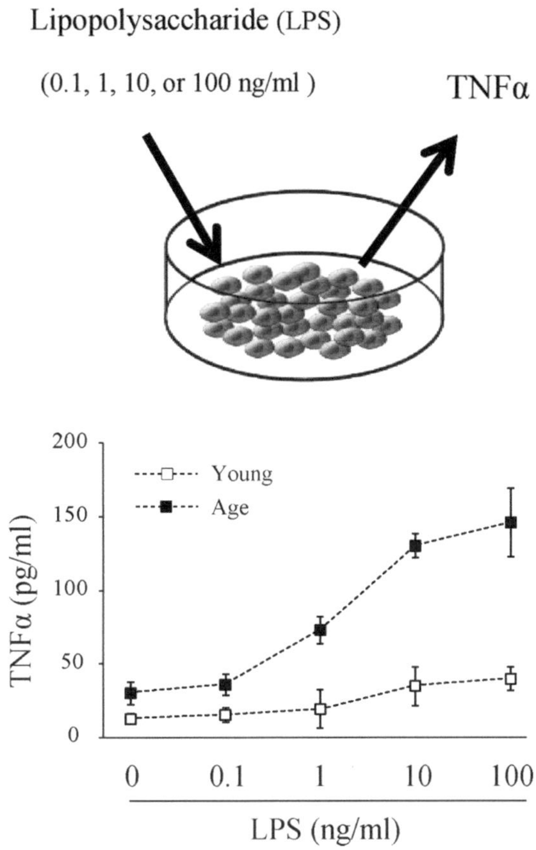

Figure 1. Microglial priming. Effects of ex vivo stimulation with lipopolysaccharide (LPS) on the cultured microglia were shown. Hippocampal microglia were isolated from either young or aged rats. Primary microglia were stimulated with 0.1, 1, 10 and 100 ng/ml or media alone, and levels of TNF-α were determined from supernatants collected 24 h later. The LPS-induced increase in TNF-α was greater in the microglia of aged rats than young. These results indicate that normal ageing may prime microglia for an exaggerated responsiveness to pro-inflammatory stimuli.

3. Treatment and prevention

Notwithstanding the fact that POCD is a common complication for geriatric patients, currently there is not any available st ment after general anaesthesia [66]. Additionally, due to the challenging nature of POCD, examples of randomized controlled studies assessing possible intervention for treating or improving POCD are scarce [2]. However, this can be addressed by studies assessing the effects of drugs on cognitive impairment after general anaesthesia. Aminophylline reduced the time necessary for postoperative cognitive recovery from sevoflurane anaesthesia, improving the ventilatory elimination of sevoflurane [67]. Meanwhile, low-dose haloperidol prophylactic treatment did not prove effective in decreasing the incidence of postoperative delirium but had a positive effect on the severity and duration [68]. A pilot, phase 2a study to evaluate the feasibility, safety and efficacy of donepezil in preventing postoperative delirium did not find significant changes in the incidence of delirium or in the days patients stayed in the hospital, although it did not rule out possible benefits [69]. In agreement with these results, Doraiswamy and collaborators [70] evaluated the effect of donepezil in treating patients with cognitive decline following coronary artery bypass graft surgery, reporting that donepezil did not improve composite cognitive performance but had enhancing effects on some aspects of memory. Meanwhile, the use of gabapentin in the treatment of postoperative pain reduced the occurrence of postoperative delirium [71].

Therefore, the lack of an effective treatment for POCD highlights the importance of the prevention. Over the past years, research efforts have been directed to identifying new strategies for preventing POCD [2]. While lidocaine administered during and after cardiac surgery failed to reduce POCD incidence, some protective effects of lower-dose lidocaine in nondiabetic subjects were found [72]. Moreover, due the anti-inflammatory action of ketamine, POCD incidence was reduced one week after cardiac surgery [73]. Meanwhile, intraoperatively intravenous administration of magnesium in cardiac surgery did not have any preventive effect over POCD [74]. Furthermore, administration of a post-cardiac surgery high dose of dexamethasone failed to reduce the risk of POCD [75], while in another study, a higher dose of dexamethasone actually increased the incidence of POCD in the early postoperative period after microvascular decompression under general anaesthesia [76]. Furthermore, resveratrol showed anti-neuroinflammation and anti-apoptosis effects attenuating the hippocampus-dependent cognitive impairment induced by isoflurane in aged mice [77]. Also, ondansetron administered postoperatively appears to have analgesic and protective effects, additionally seeming to improve the cognitive function in patients undergoing surgery under general anaesthesia [78]. When the effects of postoperative analgesia with ketoprofen on cognitive functions were investigated in aged animals, the results suggested that ketoprofen can prevent the development of surgery-associated memory deficits via its pain-relieving effects [79]. Chronic pretreatment with low doses of candesartan may elicit blood pressure-independent neuroprotective effects in POCD by decreasing hippocampal blood-brain barrier permeability and promoting resolution of neuroinflammation [47]. Further, dexmedetomidine provided neurocognitive protection, attenuating isoflurane-induced injury in rats developing brain [80]. Atorvastatin preserved the hippocampal-dependent fear response and also protected spatial memory on day seven after surgery in a mouse model of postoperative cognitive decline [81]. Aspirin-triggered resolvin D1 prevented neuronal dysfunction and cognitive decline after peripheral orthopaedic surgery in the mouse model [82].

There is considerable evidence that cognitive interventions, such as physical activity and cognitive activity, have positive effects on age-related cognitive changes as well as early-stage dementia in humans [83–89]. In addition, animal models mimicking these interventions, in which rodents were exposed to voluntary wheel running and an enriched environment, showed improvement in cognitive performance (**Figure 2**) [48, 90]. Although the mechanism of these benefits has been debated, both interventions are reported to have common positive effects on microglial number, proliferation and phenotype in the brain. In fact, preoperative cognitive intervention, a combination of physical activity and cognitive activity, has been shown to prevent the development of POCD via restoration of the pro-inflammatory phenotype in aged microglia [48]. In addition, evidence suggests that an enriched environment attenuated the surgery effects in reduction of brain-derived neurotrophic factor (BDNF) expression and neurogenesis in the hippocampus [90]. Recent time-course analysis using a rat abdominal surgery model revealed that hippocampal neuroinflammation and related microglial activation were found at 7 days after surgery, which resolved to normal levels by 14 days after surgery [48]. Therefore, the effects of pre-operative cognitive intervention may persist long enough to encompass the critical period of POCD development [48].

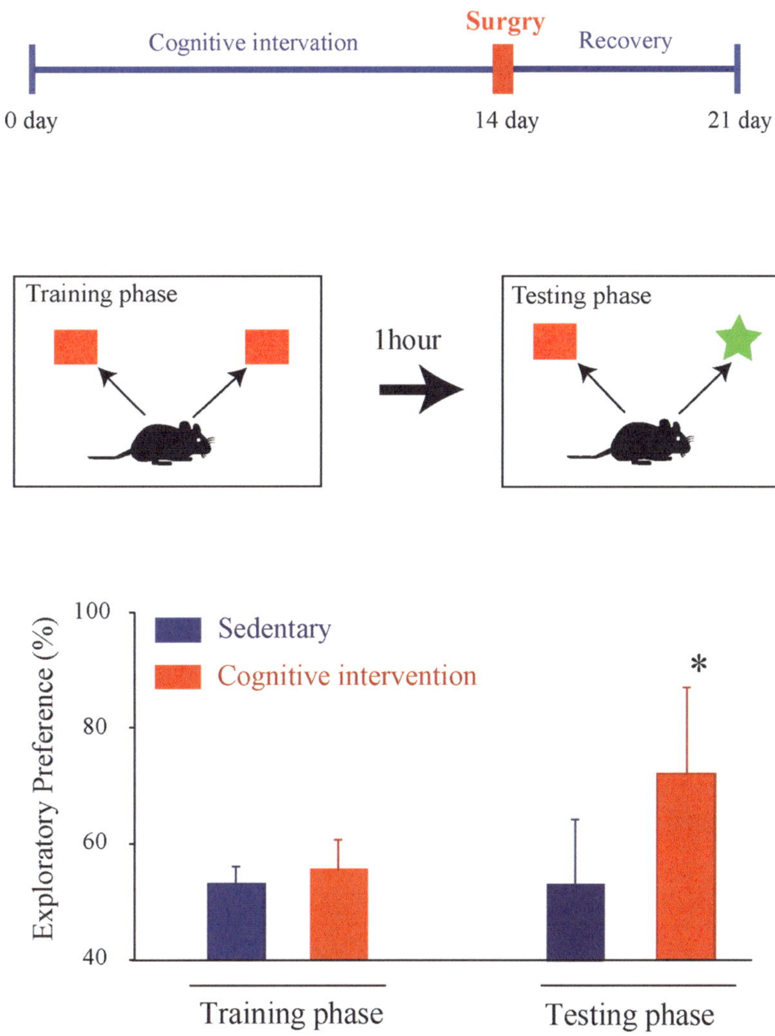

Figure 2. Effects of preoperative cognitive intervention on cognitive function assessed by novel object recognition test in aged rats. All rats were exposed to preoperative cognitive intervention or sedentary condition for 14 days following surgery (laparotomy and small intestinal manipulation) or non-surgery and allowed 7 days of recovery. Seven days after surgery, the effects of cognitive intervention on hippocampal-mediated working memory were assessed by a novel object recognition task. The sedentary rats in the aged group exhibited significantly impaired novel object recognition performance as shown by the similar amount of time spent in exploring the two objects. However, such impairment was not observed in the preoperative cognitive intervention group.

4. Concluding remarks

POCD is increasingly recognized as one of the common complications in geriatric patients despite the lack of strategy for prevention and management. Due to these limitations, preoperative management should be focused on promoting an early recognition of the patients at risk, and preventative measures should be taken from a multimodal approach comprising collaboration between the anaesthesiologist, surgeon, geriatricians and inclusion of family in the postoperative care plan in order to improve overall recovery and avoid long-term sequelae of POCD [2, 6, 10, 66]. Furthermore, it is recommended that patients at high risk for POCD should get preoperative discussion of this issue, allowing patients to make cognitively demanding decisions before surgery [2]. In addition, in line with the positive effects of cognitive interventions in both human and animal models, "pre-surgical rehabilitation" must be encouraged when possible in order to minimize the risk of POCD occurrence and its effects on overall recovery after surgery [2]. Moreover, promising new approaches such as the utilization of the relationship between neuroinflammation and miRNA expression should not be overlooked, in order to understand and discover new treatments. Deregulation of certain miRNAs may be associated with POCD development.

While both cardiac surgery and noncardiac surgery have been associated with POCD, the effects of each seem to affect different cognitive domains and in consequence may originate from different causes or mechanisms [25]. Moreover, the difficulty extrapolating the knowledge gathered through preclinical studies and animal models to human cases and the translation of these findings into therapeutic treatment for POCD points to the need for further work is needed. So far, the surgery-induced neuroinflammation processes including the microglial activation pathways seem to be the most promising therapeutic targets in the management of POCD.

Author details

Fabricio M. Locatelli and Takashi Kawano*

*Address all correspondence to: takashika@kochi-u.ac.jp

Department of Anesthesiology and Intensive Care Medicine, Kōchi Medical School, Kōchi, Japan

References

[1] Bedford PD: Adverse cerebral effects of anaesthesia on old people. Lancet. 1955; 269(6884): 259-63. doi: 10.1016/S0140-6736(55)92689-1

[2] Berger M, Nadler JW, Browndyke J, Terrando N, Ponnusamy V, Cohen HJ, Whitson HE, Mathew JP: Postoperative cognitive dysfunction: minding the gaps in our knowledge of a common postoperative complication in the elderly. Anesthesiol Clin. 2015; 33(3): 517-50. doi: 10.1016/j.anclin.2015.05.008

[3] Ageing in the Twenty-First Century. A Celebration and A Challenge New York and London. 2012. UNFPA and Help Age International. ISBN: 978-0-89714-981-5

[4] World Health Organization. World Health Statistics – Life Expectancy Increased by 5 years Since 2000, but Health Inequalities Persist [Internet] 2016. Available from: http://www.who.int/mediacentre/news/releases/2016/health-inequalities-persist/en/

[5] Jin K, James WS, Xunming J, Miriam L, Stambler I: The critical need to promote research of aging and aging-related diseases to improve health and longevity of the elderly population. Aging Dis. 2014; 6(1): 1-5. doi: 10.14336/AD.2014.1210.

[6] Yang R, Wolfson M, Lewis MC: Unique aspects of the elderly surgical population an anesthesiologist's perspective. Geriatr Orthop Surg Rehabil. 2011; 2(2): 56-64. doi: 10.1177/2151458510394606

[7] Moller JT, Cluitmans P, Rasmussen LS, Houx P, Rasmussen H, Canet J, Rabbitt P, Jolles J, Larsen K, Hanning CD, Langeron O: Long-term postoperative cognitive dysfunction in the elderly: ISPOCD1 study. Lancet. 1998; 351(9106): 857-61. doi: 10.1016/S0140-6736(97)07382-0

[8] Deiner S and Silverstein JH: Postoperative delirium and cognitive dysfunction. Br J Anaesth. 2009; 103(Suppl. 1):i41-6. doi: 10.1093/bja/aep291

[9] Monk TG, Weldon BC, Garvan CW, Dede DE, van der Aa MT, Heilman KM, Gravenstein JS: Predictors of cognitive dysfunction after major noncardiac surgery. Anesthesiology. 2008; 108(1): 18-30. doi: 10.1097/01.anes.0000296071.19434.1e

[10] De Cosmo G, Sessa F, Fiorini F, Congedo E: Postoperative cognitive disfunction in elderly patients: a frequent complication. J Anesth Crit Care Open Access. 2015; 2(2): 00048. doi: 10.15406/jaccoa.2015.02.00048

[11] Glisky EL: Changes in cognitive function in human aging. In: Brain Aging: Models, Methods, and Mechanisms. CRC Press/Taylor & Francis Boca Raton (FL) USA. 2007; 19:3-20.

[12] Wang W, Wang Y, Wu H, Lei L, Xu S, Shen X, Guo X, Shen R, Xia X, Liu Y, Wang F: Postoperative cognitive dysfunction: current developments in mechanism and prevention. Med Sci Monit. 2014; 20: 1908-12. doi: 10.12659/MSM.892485

[13] Selnes OA, Grega MA, Bailey MM, Pham LD, Zeger SL, Baumgartner WA, McKhann GM: Cognition 6 years after surgical or medical therapy for coronary artery disease. Ann Neurol. 2008; 63(5): 581-90. doi: 10.1002/ana.21382

[14] Van Harten AE, Scheeren TW, Absalom AR: A review of postoperative cognitive dysfunction and neuroinflammation associated with cardiac surgery and anaesthesia. Anaesthesia. 2012; 67(3): 280-93. doi: 10.1111/j.1365-2044.2011.07008.x

[15] Newman MF, Kirchner JL, Phillips-Bute B, Gaver V, Grocott H, Jones RH, Mark DB, Reves JG, Blumenthal JA: Longitudinal assessment of neurocognitive function after coronary-artery bypass surgery. N Engl J Med. 2001; 344(6): 395-402. doi: 10.1056/NEJM200102083440601

[16] Knipp SC, Matatko N, Wilhelm H, Schlamann M, Thielmann M, Lösch C, Diener HC, Jakob H: Cognitive outcomes three years after coronary artery bypass surgery: relation to diffusion-weighted magnetic resonance imaging. Ann Thorac Surg. 2008; 85(3): 872-9. doi: 10.1016/j.athoracsur.2007.10.083

[17] Evered L, Scott DA, Silbert B, Maruff P: Postoperative cognitive dysfunction is independent of type of surgery and anesthetic. Anesth Analg. 2011; 112(5): 1179-85. doi: 10.1213/ANE.0b013e318215217e

[18] Shaw PJ, Bates D, Cartlidge NE, French JM, Heaviside D, Julian DG, Shaw DA: Long-term intellectual dysfunction following coronary artery bypass graft surgery: a six month follow-up study. Q J Med. 1987; 62(239): 259-68. doi: http://dx.doi.org/259-268

[19] Savageau JA, Stanton BA, Jenkins CD, Frater RW: Neuropsychological dysfunction following elective cardiac operation. II. A six-month reassessment. J Thorac Cardiovasc Surg. 1982; 84(4): 595-600.

[20] Dijk D, Keizer AM, Diephuis JC, Durand C, Vos LJ, Hijman R: Neurocognitive dysfunction after coronary artery bypass surgery: a systematic review. J Thorac Cardiovasc Surg. 2000; 120(4): 632-9. doi: 10.1067/mtc.2000.108901

[21] Pugsley W, Klinger L, Paschalis C, Treasure T, Harrison M, Newman S: The impact of microemboli during cardiopulmonary bypass on neuropsychological functioning. Stroke. 1994; (7): 1393-9.

[22] Cox G, Tzioupis C, Calori GM, Green J, Seligson D, Giannoudis PV: Cerebral fat emboli: a trigger of post-operative delirium. Injury. 2011; 42(Suppl. 4): S6-10. doi: 10.1016/S0020-1383(11)70005-5

[23] Leiendecker J, Höcker J, Meybohm P, Fudickar A, Bein B: Postoperative neurocognitive function and microembolus detection in patients undergoing neck dissection: a pilot study. Eur J Anaesthesiol. 2010; 27(5): 417-24. doi: 10.1097/EJA.0b013e328336c633

[24] Qing M, Shim JK, Grocott HP, Sheng H, Mathew JP, Mackensen GB: The effect of blood pressure on cerebral outcome in a rat model of cerebral air embolism during cardiopulmonary bypass. J Thorac Cardiovasc Surg. 2011; 142(2): 424-9. doi: 10.1016/j.jtcvs.2010.11.036

[25] Hovens IB, van Leeuwen BL, Mariani MA, Kraneveld AD, Schoemaker RG: Postoperative cognitive dysfunction and neuroinflammation; Cardiac surgery and abdominal surgery are not the same. Brain Behav Immun. 2016; 54:178-93. doi: 10.1016/j.bbi.2016.02.003

[26] Fong HK, Sands LP, Leung JM: The role of postoperative analgesia in delirium and cognitive decline in elderly patients: a systematic review. Anesth Analg. 2006; 102(4): 1255-66. doi: 10.1213/01.ane.0000198602.29716.53

[27] Mc Connolly EJ: Severe pain confounds neuropsychological test performance. J Clin Exp Neuropsychol. 2000; 22(5): 633-9. doi: 10.1076/1380-3395(200010)22:5;1-9;FT633

[28] Zywiel MG, Prabhu A, Perruccio AV, Gandhi R: The influence of anesthesia and pain management on cognitive dysfunction after joint arthroplasty: a systematic review. Clin Orthop Relat Res. 2014; 472(5): 1453-66. doi: 10.1007/s11999-013-3363-2

[29] Kaneko T, Takahashi S, Naka T, Hirooka Y, Inoue Y, Kaibara N: Postoperative delirium following gastrointestinal surgery in elderly patients. Surg Today. 1997; 27(2): 107-11. doi: 10.1007/BF02385897

[30] Silbert BS, Evered LA, Scott DA: Incidence of postoperative cognitive dysfunction after general or spinal anaesthesia for extracorporeal shock wave lithotripsy. Br J Anaesth. 2014; 113(5): 784-91. doi: 10.1093/bja/aeu163

[31] Guay J: General anaesthesia does not contribute to long-term post-operative cognitive dysfunction in adults: a meta-analysis. Indian J Anaesth. 2011; 55(4): 358-63. doi: 10.4103/0019-5049.84850

[32] Mason SE, Noel-Storr A, Ritchie CW: The impact of general and regional anesthesia on the incidence of post-operative cognitive dysfunction and post-operative delirium: a systematic review with meta-analysis. J Alzheimers Dis. 2010;22(Suppl. 3): 67-79. doi: 10.3233/JAD-2010-101086

[33] Culley DJ, Baxter MG, Yukhananov R, Crosby G: Long-term impairment of acquisition of a spatial memory task following isoflurane–nitrous oxide anesthesia in rats. Anesthesiology. 2004; 100(2): 309-14.

[34] Cao L, Li L, Lin D, Zuo Z: Isoflurane induces learning impairment that is mediated by interleukin 1β in rodents. PLoS One. 2012; 7(12): e51431. doi: 10.1371/journal.pone.0051431

[35] Lin D, Zuo Z: Isoflurane induces hippocampal cell injury and cognitive impairments in adult rats. Neuropharmacology. 2011;61(8):1354-9. doi: 10.1016/j.neuropharm.2011.08.011

[36] Komatsu H, Nogaya J, Anabuki D, Yokono S, Kinoshita H, Shirakawa Y, Ogli K: Memory facilitation by posttraining exposure to halothane, enflurane, and isoflurane in ddN mice. Anesth Analg. 1993; 76(3): 609-12.

[37] Callaway JK, Jones NC, Royse AG, Royse CF: Sevoflurane anesthesia does not impair acquisition learning or memory in the Morris water maze in young adult and aged rats. Anesthesiology. 2012; 117(5): 1091-101. doi: 10.1097/ALN.0b013e31826cb228

[38] Parsons CG, Rammes G, Danysz W: Pharmacodynamics of memantine: an update. Curr Neuropharmacol. 2008; 6(1): 55-78. doi: 10.2174/157015908783769671

[39] Canet J, Raeder J, Rasmussen LS, Enlund M, Kuipers HM, Hanning CD, Jolles J, Korttila K, Siersma VD, Dodds C, Abildstrom H: Cognitive dysfunction after minor surgery in the elderly. Acta Anaesthesiol Scand. 2003; 47(10):1204-10. doi: 10.1046/j.1399-6576.2003.00238.x

[40] Scott DA, Evered LA, Silbert BSJ: Cardiac surgery, the brain, and inflammation. Extra Corpor Technol. 2014; 46(1): 15-22.

[41] McDonagh DL, Mathew JP, White WD, Phillips-Bute B, Laskowitz DT, Podgoreanu MV, Newman MF: Cognitive function after major noncardiac surgery, apolipoprotein E4 genotype, and biomarkers of brain injury. Anesthesiology. 2010; 112(4): 852-9. doi: 10.1097/ALN.0b013e3181d31fd7

[42] Hudetz JA, Patterson KM, Byrne AJ: A history of alcohol dependence increases the incidence and severity of postoperative cognitive dysfunction in cardiac surgical patients. Int J Environ Res Public Health. 2009; 6(11): 2725-39. doi: 10.3390/ijerph6112725

[43] Hudetz JA, Gandhi SD, Iqbal Z, Patterson KM, Byrne AJ, Warltier DC, Pagel PS: History of post-traumatic stress disorder is associated with impaired neuropsychometric performance after coronary artery surgery. J Cardiothorac Vasc Anesth. 2010; 24(6): 964-8. doi: 10.1053/j.jvca.2010.02.019

[44] Kalb A, von Haefen C, Sifringer M, Tegethoff A, Paeschke N, Kostova M, Feldheiser A, Spies CD: Acetylcholinesterase inhibitors reduce neuroinflammation and -degeneration in the cortex and hippocampus of a surgery stress rat model. PLoS One. 2013; 8(5): e62679. doi: 10.1371/journal.pone.0062679

[45] Cibelli M, Fidalgo AR, Terrando N, Ma D, Monaco C, Feldmann M, Takata M, Lever IJ, Nanchahal J, Fanselow MS, Maze M: Role of interleukin-1beta in postoperative cognitive dysfunction. Ann Neurol. 2010; 68(3):360-8. doi: 10.1002/ana.22082

[46] Chi H, Kawano T, Tamura T, Iwata H, Takahashi Y, Eguchi S, Yamazaki F, Kumagai N, Yokoyama M: Postoperative pain impairs subsequent performance on a spatial memory task via effects on N-methyl-D-aspartate receptor in aged rats. Life Sci. 2013; 93(25-26): 986-93. doi: 10.1016/j.lfs.2013.10.028

[47] Li Z, Cao Y, Li L, Liang Y, Tian X, Mo N, Liu Y, Li M, Chui D, Guo X: Prophylactic angiotensin type 1 receptor antagonism confers neuroprotection in an aged rat model of postoperative cognitive dysfunction. Biochem Biophys Res Commun. 2014; 449(1): 74-80. doi: 10.1016/j.bbrc.2014.04.153

[48] Kawano T, Eguchi S, Iwata H, Tamura T, Kumagai N, Yokoyama M: Impact of preoperative environmental enrichment on prevention of development of cognitive impairment following abdominal surgery in a rat model. Anesthesiology. 2015; 123(1): 160-70. doi: 10.1097/ALN.0000000000000697

[49] Hovens IB, Schoemaker RG, van der Zee EA, Absalom AR, Heineman E, van Leeuwen BL: Postoperative cognitive dysfunction: involvement of neuroinflammation and neuronal functioning. Brain Behav Immun. 2014; 38: 202-10. doi: 10.1016/j.bbi.2014.02.002

[50] Hovens IB, van Leeuwen BL, Nyakas C, Heineman E, van der Zee EA, Schoemaker RG: Postoperative cognitive dysfunction and microglial activation in associated

brain regions in old rats. Neurobiol Learn Mem. 2015; 118: 74-9. doi: 10.1016/j.nlm.2014.11.009

[51] Rosczyk HA, Sparkman NL, Johnson RW: Neuroinflammation and cognitive function in aged mice following minor surgery. Exp Gerontol. 2008; 43(9): 840-6. doi: 10.1016/j.exger.2008.06.004; doi: 10.1016%2Fj.exger.2008.06.004#pmc_ext

[52] Bluthe RM, Pawlowski M, Suarez S, Parnet P, Pittman Q, Kelley KW, Dantzer R: Synergy between tumor necrosis factor α and interleukin-1 in the induction of sickness behavior in mice. Psychoneuroendocrinology. 1994; 19(2): 197-207. doi: 10.1016/0306-4530(94)90009-4

[53] Terrando N, Monaco C, Ma D, Foxwell BM, Feldmann M, Maze M: Tumor necrosis factor-α triggers a cytokine cascade yielding postoperative cognitive decline. Proc Natl Acad Sci U S A. 2010; 107(47):20518-22. doi: 10.1073/pnas.1014557107

[54] Wilson CJ, Finch CE, Cohen HJ. Cytokines and cognition—the case for a head-to-toe inflammatory paradigm. J Am Geriatr Soc. 2002; 50(12): 2041-56. doi: 10.1046/j.1532-5415.2002.50619.x

[55] Pugh CR, Fleshner M, Watkins LR, Maier SF, Rudy JW: The immune system and memory consolidation: a role for the cytokine IL-1β. Neurosci Biobehav Rev. 2001; 25(1): 29-41. doi: 10.1016/S0149-7634(00)00048-8

[56] Murray CA, Lynch MA: Evidence that increased hippocampal expression of the cytokine interleukin-1β is a common trigger for age-and stress-induced impairments in long-term potentiation. J Neurosci. 1998;18(8): 2974-81.

[57] Jang S, Dilger RN, Johnson RW: Luteolin inhibits microglia and alters hippocampal-dependent spatial working memory in aged mice. J Nutr. 2010; 140(10): 1892-8. doi: 10.3945/jn.110.123273

[58] McAfoose J, Baune BT: Evidence for a cytokine model of cognitive function. Neurosci Biobehav Rev. 2009; 33(3): 355-66. doi: 10.1016/j.neubiorev.2008.10.005

[59] Xanthos DN, Sandkühler J: Neurogenic neuroinflammation: inflammatory CNS reactions in response to neuronal activity. Nat Rev Neurosci. 2014; 15(1): 43-53. doi: 10.1038/nrn3617

[60] Kawano T, Eguchi S, Iwata H, Yamanaka D, Tateiwa H, Locatelli FM, Yokoyama M: Pregabalin can prevent, but not treat, cognitive dysfunction following abdominal surgery in aged rats. Life Sci. 2016; 148: 211-9. doi: 10.1016/j.lfs.2016.02.021

[61] Yu X, Liu S, Li J, Fan X, Chen Y, Bi X, Liu S, Deng X: MicroRNA-572 improves early post-operative cognitive dysfunction by down-regulating neural cell adhesion molecule 1. PLoS One. 2015; 10(2): e0118511. doi: 10.1371/journal.pone.0118511

[62] Raisch J, Darfeuille-Michaud A, Nguyen HT: Role of microRNAs in the immune system, inflammation and cancer. World J Gastroenterol. 2013; 19(20): 2985-96. doi: 10.3748/wjg.v19.i20.2985

[63] Davidson-Moncada J, Papavasiliou FN, Tam W: MiRNAs of the immune system: roles in inflammation and cancer. Ann N Y Acad Sci. 2010; 1183: 183-94. doi: 10.1111/j.1749-6632.2009.05121.x

[64] Sonkoly E, Pivarcsi A: microRNAs in inflammation. Int Rev Immunol. 2009; 28(6): 535-61. doi: 10.3109/08830180903208303

[65] Soreq H, Wolf Y: NeurimmiRs: microRNAs in the neuroimmune interface. Trends Mol Med. 2011; 17(10): 548-55. doi: 10.1016/j.molmed.2011.06.009

[66] Saito S: Management of cognition as reported in Japanese historical documents and modern anesthesiology research papers. J Anesth. 2016. doi: 10.1007/s00540-016-2219-9

[67] El Tahan MR: Effects of aminophylline on cognitive recovery after sevoflurane anesthesia. J Anesth. 2011; 25(5): 648-56. doi: 10.1007/s00540-011-1190-8

[68] Kalisvaart KJ, De Jonghe JF, Bogaards MJ, Vreeswijk R, Egberts TC, Burger BJ, Eikelenboom P, Van Gool WA: Haloperidol prophylaxis for elderly hip-surgery patients at risk for delirium: a randomized k-controlled study. J Am Geriatr Soc. 2005; 53(10): 1658-66. doi: 10.1111/j.1532-5415.2005.53503.x

[69] Sampson EL, Raven PR, Ndhlovu PN, Vallance A, Garlick N, Watts J, Blanchard MR, Bruce A, Blizard R, Ritchie CW: A randomized, double-blind, placebo-controlled trial of donepezil hydrochloride (Aricept) for reducing the incidence of postoperative delirium after elective total hip replacement. Int J Geriatr Psychiatry. 2007; 22(4): 343-9. doi: 10.1002/gps.1679

[70] Doraiswamy PM, Babyak MA, Hennig T, Trivedi R, White WD, Mathew JP, Newman MF, Blumenthal JA: Donepezil for cognitive decline following coronary artery bypass surgery: a pilot randomized controlled trial. Psychopharmacol Bull. 2007; 40(2): 54-62.

[71] Leung JM, Sands LP, Rico M, Petersen KL, Rowbotham MC, Dahl JB, Ames C, Chou D, Weinstein P: Pilot clinical trial of gabapentin to decrease postoperative delirium in older patients. Neurology. 2006; 67(7): 1251-3. doi: 10.1212/01.wnl.0000233831.87781.a9

[72] Mathew JP, Mackensen GB, Phillips-Bute B, Grocott HP, Glower DD, Laskowitz DT, Blumenthal JA, Newman MF, Neurologic Outcome Research Group: Randomized, double-blinded, placebo controlled study of neuroprotection with lidocaine in cardiac surgery. Stroke. 2009; 40(3): 880-7. doi: 10.1161/STROKEAHA.108.531236

[73] Hudetz JA, Iqbal Z, Gandhi SD, Patterson KM, Byrne AJ, Hudetz AG, Pagel PS, Warltier DC: Ketamine attenuates post-operative cognitive dysfunction after cardiac surgery. Acta Anaesthesiol Scand. 2009; 53(7): 864-72. doi: 10.1111/j.1399-6576.2009.01978.x

[74] Mathew JP, White WD, Schinderle DB, Podgoreanu MV, Berger M, Milano CA, Laskowitz DT, Stafford-Smith M, Blumenthal JA, Newman MF, Fontes MA: Intraoperative magnesium administration does not improve neurocognitive function after cardiac surgery. Stroke. 2013; 44(12): 3407-13. doi: 10.1161/STROKEAHA. 113.002703

[75] Ottens TH, Dieleman JM, Sauër AM, Peelen LM, Nierich AP, de Groot WJ, Nathoe HM, Buijsrogge MP, Kalkman CJ, van Dijk D: Effects of dexamethasone on cognitive decline after cardiac surgery a randomized clinical trial. Anesthesiology. 2014; 121(3): 492-500. doi: 10.1097/ALN.0000000000000336

[76] Fang Q, Qian X, An J, Wen H, Cope DK, Williams JP: Higher dose dexamethasone increases early postoperative cognitive dysfunction. J Mol Neurosci. 2014; 52(2): 286-93. doi: 10.1007/s12031-013-0141-2

[77] Li XM, Zhou MT, Wang XM, Ji MH, Zhou ZQ, Yang JJ: Resveratrol pretreatment attenuates the isoflurane-induced cognitive impairment through its anti-inflammation and-apoptosis actions in aged mice. J Mol Neurosci. 2014; 52(2): 286-93. doi: 10.1007/ s12031-013-0141-2

[78] Papadopoulos G, Pouangare M, Papathanakos G, Arnaoutoglou E, Petrou A, Tzimas P: The effect of ondansetron on postoperative delirium and cognitive function in aged orthopedic patients. Minerva Anestesiol. 2014; 80(4):444-51

[79] Kawano T, Takahashi T, Iwata H, Morikawa A, Imori S, Waki S, Tamura T, Yamazaki F, Eguchi S, Kumagai N, Yokoyama M: Effects of ketoprofen for prevention of postoperative cognitive dysfunction in aged rats. J Anesth. 2014; 28(6): 932-6. doi: 10.1007/ s00540-014-1821-y

[80] Sanders RD, Xu J, Shu Y, Januszewski A, Halder S, Fidalgo A, Sun P, Hossain M, Ma D, Maze M: Dexmedetomidine attenuates isoflurane-induced neurocognitive impairment in neonatal rats. Anesthesiology. 2009; 110(5):1077-85. doi: 10.1097/ ALN.0b013e31819daedd

[81] Vizcaychipi MP, Watts HR, O'Dea KP, Lloyd DG, Penn JW, Wan Y, Pac-Soo C, Takata M, Ma D: The therapeutic potential of atorvastatin in a mouse model of postoperative cognitive decline. Ann Surg. 2014; 259(6): 1235-44. doi: 10.1097/SLA.00000 00000 000257

[82] Terrando N, Gómez-Galán M, Yang T, Carlström M, Gustavsson D, Harding RE, Lindskog M, Eriksson LI: Aspirin-triggered resolvin D1 prevents surgery-induced cognitive decline. FASEB J. 2013; 27(9): 3564-71. doi: 10.1096/fj.13-230276

[83] Etnier JL, Nowell PM, Landers DM, Sibley BA: A meta-regression to examine the relationship between aerobic fitness and cognitive performance. Brain Res Rev. 2006; 52(1): 119-30. doi: 10.1016/j.brainresrev.2006.01.002

[84] Williams KN: Exploring interventions to reduce cognitive decline in aging. J Psychosoc Nurs Ment Health Serv. 2010; 48(5): 42-51. doi: 10.3928/02793695-20100331-03 doi: 10.3928%2F02793695-20100331-03#pmc_ext

[85] Bherer L, Erickson KI, Liu-Ambrose T: A review of the effects of physical activity and exercise on cognitive and brain functions in older adults. J Aging Res. 2013; 2013:657508. doi: 10.1155/2013/657508

[86] Kirk-Sanchez NJ, McGough EL: Physical exercise and cognitive performance in the elderly: current perspectives. Clin Interv Aging. 2014; 9: 51-62. doi: 10.2147/CIA.S39506

[87] Van Gelder BM, Tijhuis MA, Kalmijn S, Giampaoli S, Nissinen A, Kromhout D: Physical activity in relation to cognitive decline in elderly men The FINE Study. Neurology. 2004; 63(12): 2316-21. doi: 10.1212/01.WNL.0000147474.29994.35

[88] Lytle ME, Vander Bilt J, Pandav RS, Dodge HH, Ganguli M: Exercise level and cognitive decline: the MoVIES project. Alzheimer Dis Assoc Disord. 2004; 18(2): 57-64. doi: 10.1097/01.wad.0000126614.87955.79

[89] Weuve J, Kang JH, Manson JE, Breteler MM, Ware JH, Grodstein F: Physical activity, including walking, and cognitive function in older women. JAMA. 2004; 292(12): 1454-61. doi: 10.1001/jama.292.12.1454

[90] Fan D, Li J, Zheng B, Hua L, Zuo Z: Enriched environment attenuates surgery-induced impairment of learning, memory, and neurogenesis possibly by preserving BDNF expression. Mol Neurobiol. 2016; 53(1): 344-54. doi: 10.1007/s12035-014-9013-1